VAUGHAN PUBLIC LIBRARIES

3 3288 10151646 8   JUL 2020

Your Period Handbook

D1453498

First published 2020 by
Aeon Books Ltd
118 Finchley Road
London NW3 5HT

Copyright © 2020 by Natasha Richardson

The right of Natasha Richardson to be identified as the author of this work has been asserted in accordance with §§ 77 and 78 of the Copyright Design and Patents Act 1988.

All rights reserved. No part of this publication may be reproduced, stored in a retrieval system, or transmitted, in any form or by any means, electronic, mechanical, photocopying, recording, or otherwise, without the prior written permission of the publisher.

British Library Cataloguing in Publication Data

A C.I.P. for this book is available from the British Library

ISBN-978-1-91159-774-2

Printed in Great Britain

www.aeonbooks.co.uk

YOUR PERIOD HANDBOOK

NATURAL SOLUTIONS FOR STRESS FREE MENSTRUATION

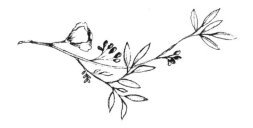

Natasha Richardson

of

FORAGE
BOTANICALS

To my ever supportive husband

Contents

My Story

I'm currently at a women's retreat, surrounded by the wilds of Snowdonia, sitting with my chai tea next to an open fire, the sound of the river in the background and the scent of nag champa incense thick in the air. I couldn't get more cliché if I tried. If I'm honest, the cliché comes naturally to me. But I feel an inner struggle. A part of me fights against the cliché because it seems to me that discovering women's mysteries and empowerment shouldn't always be wrapped in hippy packaging because it doesn't appeal to many women.

I believe there is a growing movement, a new aesthetic, which is taking the soul of feminism into a new era. One where the use of baby pink and downward pointing triangles reins supreme!

When I talk about feminism I don't just mean equal rights for men and women. The part of feminism I'm interested in is our relationship to our bodies. I think we have made great strides forward in many areas of equal rights but the education we receive about our bodies is still massively influenced by many years of patriarchy gone by.

When I was learning about medicine on my herbal medicine degree, back in 2007, the sexism that is so intermingled with the topic became more and more apparent. There is something so unquestionable about medicine. We accept its teachings under the assumption that it is the result of centuries of high quality research.

The trouble is that research wasn't always as self-reflective as it is now (and it's not great now). There are definitions and conceptualisations of fundamental facts of female and male bodies that are still shaped by the patriarchy of that time. Definitions that go so far back we've stopped questioning them. I believe it's these taken-for-granted "facts" that have the most insidious effects on us.

These definitions and concepts are so deeply set into our understanding of science they have become unquestionable. What is the origin of the word "vagina", for instance? Why do we assume women must experience pain during childbirth? Do the diagrams of our reproductive organs represent a real life woman? It is crucial that we begin to learn to question these things, to go back to the very foundations of the science of women's health and ask ourselves, is that even right?!

We must go back to the drawing board. We must be aware of the etymology of the names we use every day for ourselves, and these are just the areas we *are* taught in schools! The fact remains that there is a tonne of fabulous enlightening info we have about our bodies that we've recently discovered and don't teach.

This book will teach you everything you weren't taught at school and question all the things you were!

You don't have to be sick for your periods to be affecting your life. There are many subtle changes which menstruators experience, that can't be helped with drugs. Have you ever missed a period and wondered why? Or had a very light period and thought, where'd all the blood go? Or suddenly flooded through your underwear and trousers? Have you ever had a period come a week late following a week of emergency pregnancy tests? When our periods change it can be incredibly worrying. But, sadly, when visiting the doctor, it's pretty common to be told those changes are probably normal and there is nothing to worry about. More often than not, there is nothing they can offer you to rectify the issue.

This book is going to tell you what those changes really mean about your wellbeing, and what you can do to ensure it doesn't happen again.

We all know that there is a big difference between perfect

health and disease. But just because you don't qualify as "sick" doesn't mean you shouldn't be body-conscious and make changes to improve your wellbeing. Because, in the end, these changes, if left uncared for, can grow into illnesses like Endometriosis, Adenomyosis, Fibroids and Polycystic Ovarian Syndrome.

Sadly, getting these diagnosed can be a long uphill battle for recognition. We aren't taught in schools what symptoms are unacceptable when it comes to our periods. Menstrual wellbeing is being introduced to the syllabus in 2020! So we are left without the tools to even notice something that should be reported to a doctor. Through menstruation, birth and menopause we are treated as though our own bodies are far beyond our capability of understanding. But it is my belief that we don't have to be qualified in medicine to interpret the whispers of our body.

This book will teach you to listen to those whispers so you never have to hear it scream.

If however, you have come to this book, diagnosis in hand, screams-a-happening, I would hope this book helps you understand how managing your stress levels and mental health will help you to take the edge off your symptoms. Though the potential for healing may go way beyond just "taking the edge off", I would encourage you to find a herbalist you really click with to take it to the max.

I believe that the mind and body reflect one another, are intertwined, so it is possible that dealing with the emotional side of these illnesses has a lasting effect on the illness itself. It's certainly a pattern I have seen in countless patients in my practice. So, although this book won't speak in-depth about treating those illnesses, I have included short introductions to them to get you started, and I won't be surprised if the tips contained herein create subtle yet dramatic changes for you too.

Disease very rarely appears out of the blue. The reality is that it is often a slow journey there. Unless it is caused by a virus, an infection, or is inherited. The tricky part of inherited period problems (or those problems that start at menarche) is that the natural chaos of the first few years of menarche can make it almost impossible to tell a natural but problematic period from a period problem caused by disease. The patients I have treated as teens with menstrual problems always seem to struggle to be heard by the medical professionals. Treated as though they are simply crying wolf.

The blood tests done on the NHS could be used to try and get these people diagnosed faster. Even if my teen-patients do get a diagnosis, the only treatment offered is usually birth control. Which doesn't address the pathology but simply dictates a non-bleeding time and a bleeding time. This is usually given to women as if it fixes the underlying hormonal imbalance, but when the pill is stopped (often when conception is on the horizon) these problems return and pregnancy is very hard to come by.

We seem to be more interested in creating the impression of a period than in helping menstruators find wellbeing and true health.

There is a disconnection of periods from our bodies. As though they exist outside of us. As though, somehow, they are not integral to our being. After all, men don't have them and they're just fine!

I remember playing in the playground one day at primary school. I would have been around 8–11 years old. An older girl had brought in a teen magazine and we had been reading the questions page. There was a period question! I asked what a period was, and was told it's when you bleed between your legs. I was filled with fear and wonder all at once. Why would I bleed? Where would it come from? How could this be natural? Later that year my Mum bought me a book about adolescence that I took to school with me. My girl friends and I poured over this book, fascinated, for weeks.

When I was at school, I learnt about the cycle of hormones

4

and how they lead to pregnancy or periods. We also had a special lesson, where a woman came in and guided us through different sanitary products, and ended with her giving us a little parcel of them to go home with. I remember how exciting it was. Like we'd been welcomed into a secret club. When we left the classroom the boys wanted to know what was in our bags, but we kept it a secret, full of intrigue. We felt sophisticated, knew that if we had told them they would have acted like it was gross and made us feel worse.

I didn't learn what cervical mucous is, why my tummy seems to bloat each month, why my periods often started with brown gunk, why I felt so tired before my period, why they hurt . . . I had to teach myself all of that and because of that I felt so let down by my school for 10 years after my periods began!

I was once in sociology class at school. I must have been 17 or 18. I was daydreaming, as I often did, when a fellow student caught my eye. She looked a bit, well, green! Shortly after she slid down her chair and onto the floor, unconscious. I was agasp. Everyone surrounded her, including the teacher. Once she came back around the student simply said she'd better go home. It wasn't till she had left did someone whisper to me that she always gets bad periods. Even when they made you faint in class, we still kept the secrecy of periods sacrosanct.

FROM PAIN TO RELAXATION

I was lucky: when my periods began, they didn't cause me any trouble. They weren't particularly regular, but the pill sorted that out. It wasn't until I went to Uni that I experienced my first period problems. I can't recall when exactly the problems began, but I do remember their peak.

I had returned home for summer to work at Neal's Yard Remedies as a part time (zero hours!) sales assistant. Being on a zero hours contract meant I could go in and out of work, picking up shifts when it suited me. The work was pretty reliable, but you wouldn't know when or if it would suddenly dry up. So while it was available I tended to take all the shifts I could get. I would sometimes get a 14-day stint of work, but then I'd try to say no to work for 3 days after, so I could rest. A bit like some tube drivers in London do. Little did I know the effect it was having . . .

Our shop was in St. Pancras International train station. A busy train station, where all the shops have floor to ceiling clear glass fronts. For us it meant we were always on display. Like fish in a tank. I had come on my period and my cramps were hitting me pretty hard. I took myself behind the till point and kneeled on the floor to 1) sort leaflets and 2) hide. I knew it would pass. But after a few moments my manager approached (the most lovely motherly manager ever) and said "Hey Tash, you don't look so good". To which I replied "it's just cramps, it'll go soon". Even though I couldn't stand, let alone work, I wanted to wait it out. Then she said "I think you should go home, you look pretty green!" I stood up in shock and looked in the mirror. Sure enough, I looked green! I immediately rushed myself home in a haze of pain. I remember slouching on the train seat and trying to sleep it through. It took me an hour or so to get home. By the time I arrived, the pain had almost completely eased off. But this pattern would continue for years to come. It was also the beginning of an annoying type of pain cycle, and the thing that frustrated me most about this stabbing pain each month was that it only lasted a few hours at its peak and would soon drop down to a level I could function almost normally at. This meant that I would either have to plan things that I could easily cancel if I needed to, or leave my diary free for 3 days each month because of 2–5 hours of pain.

I tried paracetamol to manage my pain while working but found that it only took the edge off, while still making me feel extremely wishy-washy to the point where it was embarrassing to have me talking to customers because I looked like I was a million miles away! I tried herbal painkillers, but to no avail. The only thing that helped was being very drunk – again not so great while at work, though surprisingly acceptable when induced by drinking copious herbal tinctures!

It took me quite some time but I eventually figured out some things that really did help:

1. Being at home with no responsibilities
2. Heat pads
3. Evening primrose oil
4. Orgasms

I even had half a year with almost no pain, achieved while using a prescription written for me by the amazing herbalist Brittany Nickerson. Through all the trials, tribulations and never ending experiments, I came to understand that my pain wasn't the result of just my periods, it was the result of how I was living every other day of the month as well.

I remember spending one period-pain-day at home, almost totally pain free. Then someone rang me and asked me if I could do something for them. I was hit by a sudden and clear cramp. This was the day I realised that, for me to be pain free, I needed to have time alone, time where I didn't have to interact with others, and felt no demands. Because I realised it was those demands that created the kind of stress in me that leads to pain.

I started trying to take more steps to have regular chill-time in the couple of weeks preceding my period. When my hormones shifted into the luteal phase and asked me to chill out, I found that, if I did this, and took my herbs, I could be completely pain free! Even when I eventually got lazy with the herbs, so long as I managed my stress throughout the month, I could make my pain manageable.

Part One

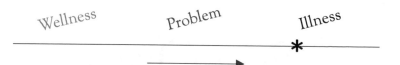

The little diagram shown here illustrates how the body moves from wellness to illness when stress affects us. With the right management in the form of herbal treatment and stress relief, we can reverse the effects back to wellness again. We will begin by talking about wellness , then cover problems and illness before coming back on overselves to wellness again (shown below).

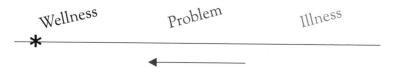

How your period works

The ever-elusive perfect period

I have heard women whisper of the perfect period. Many of us have been led to believe a 5-day bleed is optimum, when actually only around 12% of women experience this (Parry, 2005). But among "the hippies" another idea pervades, the idea that if you eat clean and live a perfectly healthy life you will achieve the ultimate, one day bleed (on a new moon).

This is, of course, a terrible myth. Terrible because all it does is give us another way to fail, another way to judge ourselves. Worse than that, it gives us a scale that is not of our own making, not attuned to us as individuals, leading us to feel that we are unwell when we aren't.

Trusting the guidance of anyone, other than yourself, to tell you what an optimum period is, is folly. Of course you'll want me to define the perfect period right now, but alas I cannot. What I can say is that when I treat patients as a herbalist I am looking for extremes as potential problems. If a period is more than 8 days, or less than 3 days in length, it is a cause for concern, but not necessarily an indicator of illness – simply a need for investigation.

Often what is more important is any sign of change. A period that goes from short to long, long to short, or short to absent is far more likely to suggest a change in health than a lifelong short bleed would.

And more important than a particular length of bleed as an indicator of health is whether that experience is causing discomfort or inconvenience to the patient, because if it's not, and they've always had periods like that, it may just be totally normal for them and their constitution.

I don't want you to aspire to a specific length; I want you to aspire to a specific comfort level. You shouldn't feel so tired before or after a bleed that normal life becomes impossible. You shouldn't experience pain that means you have to take time off work. You shouldn't be worrying about the price of sanitary care because you bleed so much.

So whilst there are "red flags" that a practitioner looks for when treating a patient with period problems, we are always open to the differences each individual patient brings, and you should be the same.

In 2016, the Eve Appeal did research which showed that only 44% of women could correctly label where the vagina is on an anatomy diagram and 60% couldn't label the labia correctly! It's quite depressing that we have such poor knowledge of the anatomical structure that has such a massive impact on our lives. The research was done to get an idea of the awareness women have of their reproductive system and how informed they are about the potential signs of the various cancers that can affect it. Considering we aren't even told that something as common as period pain is sometimes a sign of illness, I'm not surprised that signs of cancer are hardly known at all (Scott, 2016).

An interesting point to make about any anatomical diagram, however, is that they really can't capture the variety of an organic form such as the vagina. Each one is different and the illustrations are a clean cut average of those. I was totally blown away to discover that the vagina has quite an irregular shape, although if you've ever felt inside one this won't be a massive surprise! It simply isn't the tubular shape the textbooks make out. An artist was curious enough to go to the trouble of making a mould of her own and turn this beautiful shape into a book. I highly recommend going to view it at the Wellcome Collection in London. She came to understand first hand how elastic and irregular it is.

I find it interesting that the anatomical diagrams make the

vagina look like a perfect cylinder. The term vagina means "sheath", and when we come from a place where the names we have for our anatomy are from such a patriarchal viewpoint, in which vaginas are viewed, quite literally, as just the cover for their penis, you can see why anatomical diagrams, originating from this perspective look so – well – penis-like. In the past some learned individuals even hypothesised that a vagina was simply a penis that hadn't erupted from the body!

On top of this, not every woman's uterus is in the same position. Most tilt forwards, but some tilt backwards. This is called a "retroverted" uterus and it's thought to cause symptoms like period pain and poor blood flow, and even to change how you carry children. I have heard that treatments involving massage of the uterus can help this, and some patients have marvelled on its effects. But I can't recommend it outright without better evidence, so it could just be hearsay.

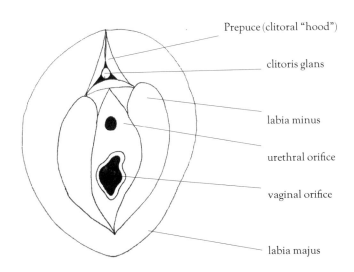

Prepuce (clitoral "hood")

clitoris glans

labia minus

urethral orifice

vaginal orifice

labia majus

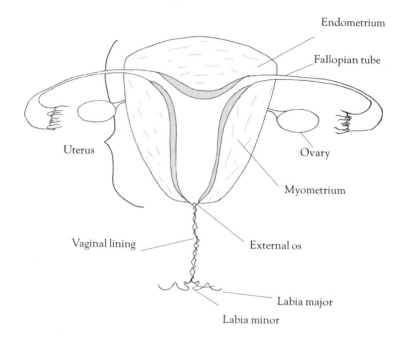

Endometrium

Fallopian tube

Uterus

Ovary

Myometrium

Vaginal lining

External os

Labia major

Labia minor

When the only images of our vulvas we're presented with are from anatomical books and porn, it's no wonder that the incidences of vaginal plastic surgery are so high, or that people go to their gynaecologist worried there is something wrong with what turns out to be their perfectly normal vulva. Labiaplasty is the fastest growing cosmetic procedure today; In 2016 45% more procedures were carried out than in 2015 (Forster, 2017).

It is our duty to engage with our own bodies, to shirk any societal ideas that this part of us is dirty or taboo to view, and to fight against the tyranny of etymology. Did you know that the word *pudendum* figuratively means a shameful part of something?

Picking up a mirror and having a look can be an empowering experience. You can also purchase speculums and look inside yourself at your cervix. At the very least it's good to look at artwork that shows a variety of real vulvas. There is also an online project called "my beautiful cervix", that shows how a real cervix changed over the course of a month.

But the reproductive system isn't just made up of our womb, vagina and vulva. It is deeply connected to 3 other endocrine glands; the hypothalamus, pituitary and ovaries. There are also 2 temporary glands that come and go with the cycle; the corpus luteum and the follicles. Following is a step-by-step outline of what is in fact a continuous cycle, unless of course a woman conceives or transitions through menopause (Trickey, 2003).

How to use herbs safely
It's very important if you have health problems that require medication that you check with a health practitioner before trying anything in this book — you need to check it'll be fine for you first.

Wellness   Problem   Illness

*

→

The Moon Metaphor

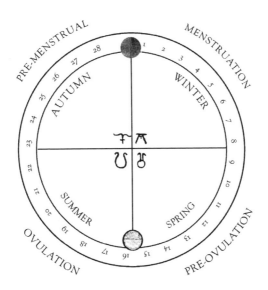

For centuries women have been associated with the moon. The moon is seen as a feminine energy, soft, gentle and nurturing. The words "menstruation" and "menses" come from the Latin menstruus, meaning "monthly", and the word "month" comes from old Norse, meaning "moon".

So you can see how intertwined menstruation and the moon are. Now, of course, that measurement of a month is written into the Gregorian calendar and doesn't resemble the actual moon cycle because it makes things a tad easier for global trade. But many women notice similarities between the moon cycle and their menstrual cycle. Sometimes, the two marry up perfectly.

It is said, by some, that all women once menstruated with the dark moon and ovulated with the full moon. I personally think this was very unlikely. But if you'd like to read more about it you can look into how to use moonlight to trigger the pineal gland and (hopefully) align with the moon again. I think it's likely that, in the past, many women had a similar cycle length and the lengths were influenced by the natural light they lived with (or lack of electric light pollution we have now).

However, each woman naturally has a slightly different cycle length and that's perfectly normal and healthy. Rather than using the moon as another measure by which we can say our periods have somehow come up short, I'd rather we use it as a wonderful metaphor to tune into our cycle more.

The moon has 4 phases: the Dark moon (or New moon), the Full moon, the Waning and the Waxing. The dark moon is a natural time of rest and hibernation each month, where we can take time to reflect and set goals for the month ahead. The full moon is the opposite of this, it is a great time to party and get out in the world. In magic this is the time to celebrate the rewards of your hard work. The waxing moon is one that is growing. It is a time where we should stay focussed on any goals set in the dark moon period to ensure they come to fruition. The waning moon is one that is getting smaller. It is a time to reflect on the goals achieved and critically analyse if that's what we really wanted, ready for fresh goals to be set in the dark moon period again.

These phases in magic and goal setting are very close to the phases we experience during the menstrual cycle. The menstrual cycle can also be split into 4 parts, as you'll see in the following pages. I hope that you'll familiarise yourself with the moon metaphor so that you can find new language to express an other-wise forgotten path of our connection and embodiment.*

---

* You can also use the seasons to understand the phases of the men-strual cycle:

Dark moon | Winter | Menstruation
Waxing moon | Spring | Preovulatory
Full moon | Summer | Ovulation
Waning moon | Autumn | Premenstrual

The Hormone Cycle

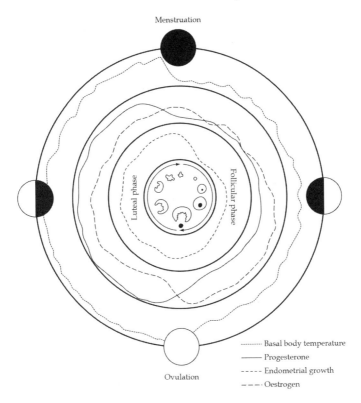

Menstruation

Luteal phase

Follicular phase

Ovulation

.... Basal body temperature

——— Progesterone

- - - - Endometrial growth

— — Oestrogen

MENSTRUAL (DAY 1–7-ish)/ DARK MOON

1. GnRH (gonadotropin releasing hormone) is released from the hypothalamus.
2. Which stimulates the release of FSH (follicle stimulating hormone) from the pituitary gland.
3. Which stimulates follicle growth.

4. Which produce oestrogen.
5. Which stimulate even more GnRH.

Physically

During menstruation the body is letting go of the unfertilised egg and endometrial lining from the previous cycle. Whilst this is occurring it is already starting to gear up for the next ovulation. The hypothalamus releases a hormone (GnRH) that tells the pituitary gland to release the follicle-stimulating hormone (FSH).

This stimulates follicles (aka immature eggs) to start to mature in the ovary on one side of the womb (ovulation alternates sides each month). Those maturing eggs make oestrogen of their own and feed back to the hypothalamus to keep providing the support it needs.

During this phase you are losing blood, of varying quantities, and this can leave you feeling drained. So be mindful of this, take it slow and eat nourishing blood building foods like raw cacao, red meat, red wine, dark leafy greens, molasses and apricots.

Emotionally

You may be feeling introspective, or hermit-like. If you can't get this space and time to yourself the outside world can get pretty tiring and annoying. Try to carve out as much me-time during your bleed as possible. Alternatively, you might be one of those people who, as soon as they bleed feel relieved, and find their energy starts to build. I was one of those people. If that's you, still try to take it easy and slowly build yourself back up into outgoing life. Try to rest just a touch longer, or spend the energy you do have on yourself, rather than prioritising others.

PRE-OVULATORY (DAY 8–14-ish)/ WAXING MOON
The hormone cycle

1. After a while the follicles begin to die off, except one. This goes on to mature into a fertile egg (ovum).
2. The rising levels of GnRH stimulate more FSH that helps the ovum to reach maturity and eventually they release LH (luteinising hormone) as well.

Physically

After a few days most of those follicles start to die off, except the one that will go on to be the egg for that cycle. Once a peak surge of FSH is reached the pituitary gland releases luteinising hormone that triggers ovulation itself.

Emotionally

Your energy has built up since you bled and this is when you'll start to want to go out and socialise again. It's a good time to make plans, and communicate anything to your loved ones that you discovered during the menstrual or premenstrual phase.

OVULATORY (DAY 15–21-ish)/ FULL MOON
The hormone cycle

1. The LH stimulates the release of the matured egg (ovulation), leaving behind a corpus luteum (surrounding material which had held the ovum).

Physically

The egg is released from the ovary and starts its journey down the fallopian tube. The body has the next 24–48 hours to fertilise that egg or pregnancy won't occur that month. The egg leaves behind the capsule that it grew in; this is called the corpus luteum.

The corpus luteum will release its own progesterone for the next few days in the hopes that pregnancy does occur. This supports the endometrial lining for the next few days.

Emotionally

This is the peak of your energy for most of you. It's also when you're feeling most sexy and sociable. Make the most of it by going out or booking in those important meetings. You will feel confident and be at your best for communication. Words will flow freely from your mouth. You'll feel like you've had some of the luck potion, Felix Felicis, from Harry Potter!

PRE-MENSTRUAL (DAY 22–28-ish)/ WANING MOON

The hormone cycle

1. After ovulation occurs levels of FSH and LH drop suddenly, and the corpus luteum starts to release its own progesterone.
1. Lowering levels of LH, FSH and oestrogen lead to the shedding of the endometrial lining (should impregnation not occur).
2. Eventually this drop in hormones contributes to GnRH being released by the hypothalamus, and the cycle begins again (Trickey, 2003).

Physically

It takes a little while for the body to realise ovulation hasn't occurred, and as the corpurs luteum uses up its resources and disappears, progesterone takes a nosedive, initiating menstruation.

Emotionally

It's normal to feel easily irritated and moody during this time because your energy reaches a natural low point. Communication skills are at their lowest but your instincts are heightened. If there is a contradiction between your instincts and what you are able to do this causes friction and irritability, which you're not very good at expressing in a considered way. It tends to all come tumbling out in angry or tearful outbursts instead. To be on the safe side, we usually pick a tiny, insignificant pet-hate to lay into so we can express the feelings without actually making any real progress. It's pretty impressive. I have found that if I'm able to actually have downtime to relax, lessen my work load and eat well then my irritability and tearfulness just doesn't occur. I implore you to experiment with using this phase to transition into a time of self-reflection and solitude.

We often think of hormonal illness occurring within the ovaries and womb only, but actually you can see how the health of your pituitary and hypothalamus are integral to good hormonal balance. In fact, the whole endocrine system is involved. Assuming, therefore, that altering oestrogen levels will be the cure of all your ailments is naïve if the hypothalamus is the one really struggling. You might be able to help the symptoms for a while but you haven't dealt with the cause. I have found that if you don't deal with the cause the body will eventually come to express that disturbance in a different way instead until you do!

If you look at the diagram on the following page you can see how the hormonal levels peak and dip. Steps 1–6 are called the follicular phase of the cycle, and everything from steps 7–9 is called the luteal phase. This is on account of the follicles which grow in the first part and the corpus luteum which is present in the last part (Meisami, Macey, and Kapit, 1997).

It took me years to really understand the hormone cycle without having to revise it in a text book. So don't feel bad if it sounds way too complicated. But this is the chapter you should return to when I use this jargon later on in the book. Usually, when you can see a practical application for this information, you're much better able to assess what's happening with your body.

Cycle day

Moon phase

Season

Basel body temp

Ovarian cycle

Hormone levels

Endrometrial lining

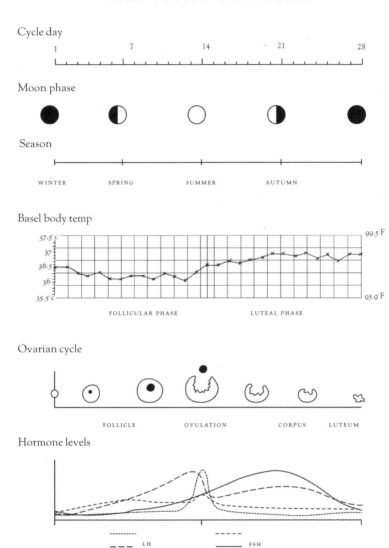

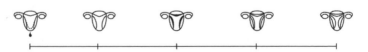

24

For instance, if your period is made of endometrial tissue you can see that having a light period would mean you didn't build up much endometrial tissue. This can happen for lots of different reasons but at least you have one more piece of the puzzle by understanding that.

Another example is Endometriosis. This is an illness where the endometrial lining grows in places other than inside the womb. It is caused by elevated oestrogen levels and often results in heavy, and painful, periods.

Often a period problem like pain can be caused by a number of things and it's important to understand what the cause is if you want to treat it hormonally. But because I don't expect you to self-diagnose, and couldn't possibly teach you how to do that here, I've carefully selected advice that enables you to improve symptoms without necessarily curing the hormonal cause. However, if the problem isn't all too serious you may find that the advice offered in this book does exactly that.

The Hormones

There are a few hormones that will get repeatedly mentioned throughout the book, and which I'd like to explain in depth below. I hope that you'll find my explanation more engaging than those in science textbooks you may have read at school on the topic.

Sadly the word "hormones" has become grossly misused in modern culture, and used as a catch-all word to explain or excuse any unpleasant emotional outbursts on the part of a woman. There also seems to be a lot of confusion around them, to the point that when women tell me they'd like to know more about their hormones, what they actually mean by this varies massively. Some want to know why they lose hair after giving birth; others want to know if they're perimenopausal. We tend to see these "hormones" as being centred on the ovaries and womb. But in reality our hormones are chemical messengers that travel throughout the body, from many endocrine glands, and are not unique to just women. They govern things such as our bone density, moods, skin health, libido, heart health and more. Men could also use the phrase "sorry I'm a bit hormonal today" and be completely correct!

In the past we have strongly associated testosterone with a masculine identity and oestrogen with a feminine one. Biologically speaking they do define our sex to a large extent, however we've come to realise that they do not necessarily define our gender identity. The key information that I think people often skim over or forget is that both men and women need both testosterone and oestrogen for proper health. Either sex would be lost without their counterpart hormone.

If, after reading this chapter, you identify yourself as having a hormone imbalance, I would HIGHLY recommend that you go to your GP for blood tests to confirm your suspicions before looking into herbs or supplements to fix your supposed "testosterone excess", since it's incredibly hard to self-diagnose, and even harder to find natural remedies that will work without guidance from someone with experience. The remedies and lifestyle changes I talk about later in the book are safe to use without needing to know what hormone is the culprit of your symptoms. They have been carefully chosen to support overall wellbeing, without manipulating the hormones directly.

TESTOSTERONE (A TYPE OF ANDROGEN, THE "MALE" HORMONE GROUP)

Normally viewed as the male hormone, testosterone is crucial to women as well. This hormone is the apogee of the qualities we have come to define as "masculinity". It creates muscles, strong bones, and raises libido. But it also makes a person feel assertive, positive and confident. When men and women are too low on this hormone they can experience depression and anxiety. Of course, it is higher in most men than women and gives rise to the male hair growth pattern, testicles and voice dropping during puberty.

Women need testosterone along with other "male" androgens, so they can be converted to the "female" hormones known as Estrogens. This conversion is managed by the sex hormone binding globulin (SHBG) to ensure there is always a balance. Usually testosterone and oestrogen are viewed as opposites, in that when one is high the other is low, and vice versa. But in reality, because they are just one of a few male or female hormones there are ways that the body may have both high oestrogen and testosterone at the same time! So don't go assuming that if you've got high levels of one the other will be relatively low (although this is, *usually*, the case).

When testosterone is out of balance these symptoms may occur:

Oily skin

Whiskers on the chin /
  upper lip or nipple

Acne

Sagging skin

Fatigue

Anxiety

Infertility

Depression

Weight gain

PCOS

Menstrual irregularity

Missed periods

Cessation of ovulation

Low libido

Things that would cause testosterone imbalance are:

Low-fat diets

Stress

Depression

Toxins from the environment

Not enough exercise

Trauma

Menopause

OESTROGEN (PART OF THE "FEMALE" HORMONE GROUP ESTROGENS)

Oestrogen is famously associated with the process of being "female". Without it, you'd struggle to define yourself as a woman, biologically speaking. It creates the "womanly" body changes of puberty, such as bigger hips, breasts, cervical mucous, female hair growth pattern and more. It's natural to think the ovaries produce these but actually oestrogen is also made by the adrenal glands and fat tissue; an important fact to keep in mind when dealing with hysterectomies and menopause.

When oestrogen is in good balance it has a role to play in how we utilise fats, and therefore protects the heart. It supports bone growth and bone density, and has a large part to play in ovulation. It also helps us feel communicative, outgoing and positive about life.

When oestrogen is out of balance these symptoms may occur:

Mood swings
Irregular or painful periods
Endometriosis (inflammatory disease where tissue grows where it shouldn't)
Depression
Breast tenderness
Weak bones that are easily fractured (osteopaenia or osteoporosis)
Vaginal dryness
light periods
Menopausal symptoms like hot flushes, fatigue, and night sweats
PMS

Things that would cause oestrogen imbalance are:

Oestrogens from the environment (e.g. plastics)
Insulin resistance (diabetes)
High sugar intake
Poor liver function
Genetic disease
Thyroid imbalance
Anorexia
Chemotherapy
Hysterectomy
Menopause
The contraceptive pill

PROGESTERONE

Progesterone is the nurturing, "motherly" hormone. It helps us to create the perfect bedding for a fertilised egg to nestle in and goes on to sustain a pregnancy until its natural conclusion at birth. It also helps us feel chilled out and laid back about life!

When progesterone is out of balance these symptoms may occur:

Scant periods
Short luteal phase
Irregular periods
Fatigue
Low libido
Weight gain
Anxiety
Depression
Headaches or migraines
Hot flushes

Things that would cause progesterone imbalance are:

Thyroid imbalance
Stress
Insulin imbalance
(aka diabetes)

Polycystic ovarian
syndrome (PCOS)
Long-haul flights and shift
work (disturbance to the
circadian rhythm)

LUTEINISING HORMONE (LH)

This lesser known hormone is crucial to fertility. Its main function is to increase body temperature and tell the body to keep up with producing progesterone. It is created by a temporary gland called the *Corpus luteum*, which is the material left behind when the mature egg bursts from its gooey container in ovulation.

If you don't have any luteinising hormone in your bloodstream after around day 14 of your cycle it's probably because you didn't ovulate. The reasons why you didn't ovulate can be many, and for this reason it's worth knowing what the hormone does, and therefore what low levels might mean on a test. It's one of the indicators for infertility. Conversely, if you have high levels of LH outside of the expected time for ovulation it's likely you've started the menopausal shift.

When LH is out of balance these symptoms may occur:

Irregular periods
No periods
Menopausal symptoms e.g.
hot flushes, night sweats,
dry vagina

Fatigue
Weight loss
Weakness
Decreased appetite

Things that would cause LH imbalance are:

PCOS
Pituitary disorder

Stress
Early menopause

Low BMI (e.g. anorexia) Menopause
High exercise   Hysterectomy

FOLLICLE STIMULATING HORMONE (FSH)

Another not-so-well-known hormone, FSH is generated by the pituitary gland, and it stimulates the ovaries to make follicles (immature eggs). This happens during the first half of the menstrual cycle, and gives that half of the menstrual cycle the name "follicular phase".

When the FSH is out of balance these symptoms may occur:

Poor sense of smell Decreased appetite
No periods   Menopausal symptoms e.g.
Fatigue   hot flushes, night sweats,
Weight loss   dry vagina

Things that would cause a FSH imbalance are:

Ovarian failure   Pituitary disorders
Early menopause Hypothalamus disorders
Menopause   Kallman's Syndrome

CORTISOL

Cortisol is the most famous stress response hormone, produced by the adrenal glands following stimulation from the hypothalamus. But just because it's associated with stress doesn't make it all bad. It energises us when we need it most. But we do tend to need it a lot in our society, and it's when it's over-used that problems occur.

When cortisol is out of balance these symptoms may occur:

Insomnia   Increased cholesterol
Lowered immunity Irregular periods

Fatigue
Depression
Anxiety
Weight gain (especially
   round the middle) or
   significant weight loss
   when cortisol is low
Poor concentration
Headaches

Painful periods
PMS
Infertility
Poor memory
Easy bruising
Acne
High blood pressure
Irritability

Things that would cause cortisol imbalance are:

Stress
Adrenal fatigue
Cushing's syndrome
   (high cortisol)
Corticosteroids

Addison's disease
   (low cortisol)
Pituitary gland disorders
High circulating oestrogen

Adrenal fatigue is a syndrome, and a collection of symptoms. It is not an accepted medical diagnosis and it isn't truly a disease. In that sense it's very similar to PMS. It's just a neat way of describing a collection of symptoms and therefore can't be tested for on a blood test.

It doesn't necessarily show up as low cortisol on a blood test. True adrenal insufficiency is called Addison's disease. But adrenal fatigue is a very useful term to help us understand a state of sub-par health and how to support ourselves through it. The symptoms include: fatigue, anxiety or depression, body aches, weight loss, poor sleep, poor concentration, and low blood pressure.

If you think you are dealing with adrenal fatigue this book is full of my own personal stories struggling with this state, which I hope you will find helpful.

THYROXIN

Is just one of a few hormones the thyroid produces. All of these hormones work in close harmony with each other to help us maintain good energy, metabolism, hair, skin and nail quality and our temperature. I see it as a "hormone of wellbeing".

When thyroxin is out of balance these symptoms may occur:

Irregular periods
Miscarriage
Infertility
Fatigue
Brain fog
Coldness
Weight change
High cholesterol
Constipation
Goitre (swelling in the throat)
Drooping eyelids
Low basal body
temperature during the
first 5 days of the cycle
Hair loss

Things that would cause thyroxin imbalance are:

Long-term stress
Shift work or many
long-haul flights
Poor liver function
Grave's disease
Immune problems such
as Hashimto's disease
Toxins from the
environment

The trouble with testing for thyroid problems (on the NHS in particular) is that they tend to only look at T3. These are the active forms of thyroid hormone, and if one of these is low then a drug replacement of those hormones is given. However, there are other hormones further up in the production line that need to be assessed as a potential cause. T4 needs to be converted into T3 to be most useful. If this isn't happening you can take all the thyroxine (T4) in the world and you won't get your best thyroid function level (Kumar & Clark, 2016). There are also hormones called anti-T3 and anti-T4, which break down and deactivate those hormones. Without testing for those you could be taking thyroxine but never actually be able to use it. These problems don't just occur in the thyroid gland, they can happen further up the ranks in the pituitary or hypothalamus, so looking just only way down the line at the thyroid can often miss the cause, and sadly lead to ultimately untreated thyroid problems.

Keeping Track

The most important thing you can do for your menstrual well-being is start to keep track. Without knowing when your last period was or how long it lasted you can't know for sure how to compare it with the next. There are many other symptoms which may turn out to be monthly, which you'll need to record in order to remember that, like migraine. In fact, research has shown that just keeping track can reduce symptoms as they reveal themselves as part of your monthly pattern, not a random mallady. The most in-depth precise way to track your cycle is FAM, but I'm not going to teach it here because you can't use hormonal contraceptives with it; instead I'll explain why I like it and give you a tracking method you can use, regardless of your contraceptive choice.

THE FERTILITY AWARENESS METHOD

Unless you've been trying to get pregnant you probably won't have heard of the fertility awareness method. It uses bodily signs like your waking temperature, cervical mucous and cervix position to tell when you are ovulating. But it's having a revival with the invention of fertility tracking apps.

I have chosen not to include the ins and outs of the method in this book as I don't want to put a lot of weight on the method when this book should feel open to all women choosing any contraceptive method. If you find that I've piqued your interest though, you can learn the method on my online course. You may even be lucky enough to find a FAM practitioner in your area. Lots work privately but some are on the NHS. I had a practitioner who could teach me the method when I was at school in New Cross (London)! I had no idea how lucky that was, I just assumed it was available to everyone. I really recommend working with someone you can get personal advice from because everyone's charts are different and it's normal for you to feel very critical of your own when you start charting. It can take a while to be able to see what's your norm, and what's unusual for you. Having someone there to hold your hand and answer any personal questions is crucial. After a year or so of charting diligently you'll probably find you don't need to keep charting in order to know where you are in your cycle. Like myself, I didn't even start to take my temperature again when I wanted to get pregnant, I just hedged my bets based on my symptoms and turned out I was right!

It'll be very tempting to use one of the new fancy apps that claim they can tell you when you're ovulating, but I have quite a few criticisms of them below. I would highly recommend going with pen, paper and practitioner over them. At least until you get a good instinct for your own cycles.

I used to feel like I was vulnerable to becoming pregnant. As if my fertility was a weakness that would be exploited by sperm. I felt like it could happen at any time, and my life would be forever changed. I needed to shut that part of me down. I needed to know it was all "under control".

So I took the contraceptive pill diligently. But as I entered the world of natural living I analysed everything that I did, from the food I ate, to the beauty products I used. So, when a friend told me she didn't use hormonal contraception, I was intrigued, but also scared. I assumed she must be in a place in her life where an accidental pregnancy was no big deal. You can imagine how shocked I was to find that even the NHS website rated this method as more effective than male condoms. In fact, male condoms were rated as 98% effective, caps and diaphragms 92-96%, the pill as more than 99% and the fertility awareness method (the one she was using) rated as up to 99% effective.

Why was it that this method was as, or more effective than all the others but I had never heard of it? With all the other methods I still felt vulnerable. I still felt ultimately out of control. All it took was a minor malfunction in the contraceptive I was using. I also felt somewhat in the hands of the gynaecologist who provided the contraception. It was like my vagina was a mysterious cave that only they could possibly understand, and I should take their advice because how could I possibly understand it better than they did?

Cue FAM (Fertility Awareness Method)

It's hard for me to describe how discovering FAM felt. Its effects on me are so far-reaching, so all-encompassing. How can I summarise such a thing? I've chosen two of the most pertinent socio-political things it has changed in me to try to hint at how amazing it has been.

1. Should we always be switched on, energetically and sexually?

The pill made me feel sexually available 100% of the time, with no baby side effects. But it robbed me of any natural downtime, any natural alone time, any natural me-time. It made me ask; if women are expected to always be sexually available and socially extroverted no wonder all the men feel like that too. No wonder we, as a society, work and work till it makes us sick. No wonder we beat ourselves up over sick days off. No wonder we feel a sense of pride when explaining that we're just so busy busy busy.

2. How does removing women from their natural cycles remove us from the natural world?

I was robbed of my natural cyclisity. When half the population (women) lose connection to their natural ebb and flow of extroversion and introversion, fertility and subfertility, energy and rest, is it really surprising we are also losing connection with the bigger cycles, like the seasons, or even just night and day? I live in a country that thrives on working all the time.

In London, the night tube has been introduced. It operates 24/7 on two of the train lines on a Friday and Saturday. Great for people going out in town, as many do. Most people think it's a wonderful thing. I, personally, like it just the way it is, but it's only a matter of time before they roll it across all the train lines every day of the week. I fear this is just the beginning of a 24/7 London. Another reason to expect people to work through the night. Which is incredibly bad for our health.

I'm not saying that the way we approach sexuality is the start of the modern world's problems. It is likely just a part of it. One that, I know, I can help change. I know FAM won't be a practical contraceptive method for many women for a variety of reasons. But while it's simply not being taught in our schools, we can't fathom how many more women there are in the world who, like me, think it's the best thing ever, a technique that has changed my life for the better. It can also be used to help you get pregnant and help you understand your hormone imbalances if you have an illness which affects them.*

---

* NOTE: After using this method successfully for over 10 years as a contraceptive (with no close calls) I am very happy to say I was able to use the method to conceive in the very first month of trying. I believe this to be because I knew when I was ovulating (no tests required I could just tell from my signs and symptoms), because I've spent years looking after my fertility and wellbeing and, lastly, I was lucky enough to not be afflicted with some sort of undiagnosed fertility problem.

LEARNING FAM (AND THE DANGER OF APPS)

One of these apps has gone so far as to become registered as a contraceptive called Natural Cycles. Despite this, it has been criticised by the Advertising Standards Agency in the UK for making misleading claims in their adverts as to its efficacy (Davis, 2018).

I love a good app as much as the next millennial but I've been practicing fertility awareness for a lot longer than the apps have existed and I have my concerns.

While the app is 93% effective, the pen and paper method I learnt is up to 99% effective (NHS, 2017)! I've tried these apps and have yet to find one which can tell me when I'm ovulating more accurately than I can for myself.

It's Missing 2 Fundamental Pieces of Info

What I don't like about the app is that it doesn't actually teach you FAM, it just takes your waking temperature and average cycle length to dictate 10 days in which you shouldn't have sex, making you reliant on the algorithm. Whereas, FAM teaches you how to interpret the signs and symptoms of your body until you don't need a chart. The app omits recording cervical mucous and cervix position. Which reduces its effectiveness (Knight, 2017).

It only uses your waking temperature. Taking your waking temperature can only ever tell you *after* you've ovulated because your temp needs to rise by 0.2 degrees for 3 consecutive mornings. Natural Cycles is being quite cautious by allowing 10 days for the fertile window when there is only a 5% chance sperm will survive more than 4.4 days and a 1% chance sperm will live more than 6.8 days in a fertile woman (Ferreira-Poblete, 1997).

Recently the app was reported to authorities in Stockholm

after 37 women seeking abortions were discovered to have been users of the app (Murphy, 2018). But maybe they fit inside the 7% of "error" that their research predicts even with perfect use. We can't know unless someone tells us how many women were using it who didn't get pregnant in correlation with those 37 who did.

The research was done by the company themselves

However, the research on its effectiveness was done by the app creators themselves. Research is expensive and only worthwhile if the research can be used to make money in the end. So I'll remain skeptical until an independent study is done. After all, drug companies who conduct their own research aren't exactly known for their impartial results.

FAM RECOMMENDED RESOURCES

My favourite books for learning the fertility awareness method are (in order of preference):

1. *Honouring our Cycles* by Katie Singer
2. *Taking Charge of Your Fertility* by Toni Weschler
3. *The Complete Guide to Fertility Awareness* by Jane Knight (a definitive reference book)

You can find a practitioner of FAM here:
fertilityuk.org/find-a-clinic/

You can buy a beautiful charting manual here:
penandpaperfertility.com

Or download sheets for free from Katie Singer's website here:
gardenoffertility.com/fertilitycharts.shtml

My course:
foragebotanicals.teachable.com

HOW TO CHART YOUR CYCLE

Although I'm an advocate for FAM it's quite full-on and not always practical. To benefit from this book, I recommend the following method of tracking as the bare minimum, and learn FAM as maximum. I'd recommend that you at least record a handful of symptoms in your diary, correlating it with the day of your cycle. The things I'd record are:

Your emotions
Energy levels
Sleep quality
Stress levels
Any symptoms you associated with your period that you want to track, like sore boobs for instance.

Just write down how good or bad they were on a 1–5 scale so it's easy to see if things got better or worse. I know someone who also attributed a colour to the number rating.

This made it very quick to see whether it had gotten hotter or colder. This will help with the connection you have with your body, and help you be able to track what changes in lifestyle, diet or herbs are making the real impact. You can read more about recording things in the "How to choose herbs that are right for you" section in the second part of the book.

But what if I use the contraceptive pill?

All the "normality" and wellness we've spoken of so far applies to a natural hormone cycle. Something many of you won't be having. When I was a teen I was led to take the contraceptive pill shortly after my periods began, as though it were a right of passage, the mature adult thing to do. I didn't question that for years, and this may be the start of you questioning your use of it.

So, although I'm not anti-pill, I've included the following info because I know it will answer many of your questions.

THE PILL

It's not infrequent for someone suffering with period problems to be offered the contraceptive pill by their doctor to "regulate their periods". This is a falsehood and I'd like to explain why, as I often end up treating patients after they've come off the pill, only to realise all the problems they had before are still there.

There are a few different types of contraceptive pills: progesterone only, oestrogen only and a combination of the two (the combined pill). By giving the same dose of hormones each day the body is tricked into leaving the natural cycle, and essentially thinks it's on the same day of the cycle every day. Often people say it's like being pregnant, but it's really not as hormones do not stay the same every day, they steadily rise over the course of pregnancy.

If it's an oestrogen only pill it thinks it's somewhere in the follicular phase each day. If it's a progesterone only pill it thinks it's somewhere in the luteal phase. When you take a 7-day break from taking your pill each month you start to bleed. This isn't caused by the fact you ovulated and then didn't conceive. It's just a side effect of the immediate removal of hormones from the system. The only reason you have this break in-between pills is because the people who designed the pill in the 1960s thought women would find it unacceptably unnatural to stop their periods altogether. Nowadays we aren't so concerned about this, as contraceptive pills are taken without breaks to get through a holiday without the inconvenience, or contraceptive injections are used which stop the periods for months on end. It's quite interesting how different our opinions are now, compared to that of the woman of the 1960s. Perhaps we've all been taking the pill for so long we don't see the appeal of a natural cycle anymore.

So when you take a contraceptive pill to "regulate the period", you're actually producing a totally different hormone "cycle", one of consistency, then intentional elimination on a recurring basis. Not the natural cycle of a repetitive build and decline, which works like a wave. When you decide to stop taking it, it's no surprise that whatever hormone issue there was before is often just waiting to come back again. Contraceptive pills don't balance your hormones; they just give the impression of a regular period, and act as a pause button for your period problems, if you will.

For those who want the chemical understanding of what the pill does, here it is:

"Oral contraceptives (OCs) function primarily by acting on the hypothalamus to cause diminution of gonadotropin-releasing hormone (GnRH) secretion, and consequently that of luteinizing hormone (LH) and follicle stimulating hormone (FSH). The ovary is no longer stimulated and produces only a slight amount of estradiol. GnRH secretion rapidly resumes when OCs are terminated, but the resting ovary is not always able to respond immediately to hypothalamic stimulation. A sufficient level of estradiol must be secreted before ovulation can ensue." (Wyss & Bourrit, 1986)

COMING OFF IT

After months of cystitis and thrush, I gave up the pill for good. I was about 19 at the time and I'd heard from a friend that it might be the cause, and they were right. So I started using my first ever hormone-free contraceptive (aside from condoms): the fertility awareness method (FAM).

But despite my personal experience I still don't feel that the pill is the work of the devil and certainly don't preach against its use. It is clear to me that the change of hormones, ph and microflora the pill created led to my cystitis-thrush pattern, even though I had used it for many years before that without any problem! I don't know why my body changed its response to a pill I'd been using for years, but it just happened to coincide with me learning more and more about the natural female cycle and wanting to be a part of it again.

I'm not writing this section because I want you to come off the contraceptive pill, but because many reading this will already be wondering about coming off it, and I think information on the topic is woefully riddled with superstition.

How long till the pill wears off?

Most women will start having periods again within 3 months of stopping the pill. If you don't have one within 6 months of stopping the pill it's called post-pill amenorrhea and affects about 0.2–3% of women. 1 in 3 women will have a period within a month of stopping the pill and 93% within 3 months. The variability between women on how quickly their periods return will depend on things such as their liver function, exposure to external toxins, and the relative balance of their other hormones (Wyss & Bourrit, 1986).

It seems that often women blame the pill for their periods going awry after stopping it. But the reality is that, sadly, the pill is overprescribed for "regulating" the cycle in the first place. So when the pill is stopped the old irregular cycles return because the pill doesn't address the underlying hormonal imbalance which led to the irregularity, it simply suppresses ovulation and gives the impression of a regular cycle instead.

Although taking the pill may have contributed to whatever symptoms you're experiencing it's near on impossible to even prove it is the cause. So while I think it's great for us to stay open to the possibility, I don't think it's particularly scientific to lay the blame on the pill as that is just plain ol' biased behaviour without the evidence to back it up.

What can I take to regulate my cycles after the pill?

You shouldn't need to do anything really. In fact, it's probably best to avoid anything that might change your hormones, otherwise you'll never know what your periods are naturally like. It's fairly common that women feel that the pill lingers in their body for days or months after it has been stopped. But you wouldn't need to take it every day for it to work if it was actually in your system for that long.

I'd argue, on that logic, that the drugs are out of your body within 24 hours. But because the ovaries have been suppressed for a while it can take time for them to be stimulated again, especially if the pill was given so early in life that the ovaries never really got a chance to grow the receptors they need to be tickled into action.

The trouble with side effects

If you've ever actually read the information pamphlet that comes with your contraceptive pill you will have noticed a long list of potential side effects. It's perfectly normal that taking something that changes the natural course of your body so dramatically should have side effects; the trouble is that while you're taking it, it's very difficult to know if the pill is causing the effect or something else. If only you had a twin, experiencing

your exact same life but who wasn't taking the pill, to compare with.

The other problem is that we take the pill for so long that, if
anything changes in our health, it's natural to ignore the pill as
the potential cause. That's what I did. The only surefire way of
knowing the pill is the cause is to stop taking it. That can seem
like an extreme measure, but I would really recommend it.

But of course, get prepared with other non-hormonal contraceptives before taking the dive. You can always go back on
a different type of contraceptive pill once you've figured out
the cause of the problem. This isolates the variables as much
as possible, giving the clearest results.

Hormone-free contraceptive options

Let's not pretend that because you stop taking the pill you want to get pregnant, so here are your hormone-free alternatives.

I don't know about you but I have been brainwashed into thinking using anything less than the contraceptive pill or depo-provera injection is irresponsible contraception. But no contraceptive is 100% effective.

I decided many moons ago that it was actually more responsible to have 2–3 contraceptives between you and pregnancy if you really don't want to have babies. My first line of defence was the pill, my second line was a condom (also crucial to avoid infections) and my third line was the morning-after pill for any potential mishaps with the condom.

That probably all seems a bit mental. But, I'm sorry to say that most young people have given up condoms believing that the pill is all they need. Of course, this is leading to a massive increase in sexually transmitted infections. We have brilliant drugs to treat most infections but I don't think young people are being taught about the potential long-term effects on their fertility from being repeatedly infected.

Maybe you'll decide to layer your contraceptives as I once did. But I totally respect if you don't, it's not exactly convenient. But perhaps we do need to return to the days where sexual relationships were more considered than they are now. For the sake of everyone's physical and mental health.

THE CONDOM

Condoms have sadly seen a dramatic drop in popularity among 16–24 year-olds recently, one that is increasing the rates of

Gonorrhoea and Chlamydia again. This age group accounts for 55% of those STIs, with 47% of them saying they have had sex with a new partner without a condom (Greenfield, 2017). When I was at school (not very long ago, let's face it) condoms were promoted as practically a necessity when it came to sex.

It's important that we get to the bottom of why they are turning away from this form of contraception, as prevention is always better than cure. I think it's possible that the cautiousness has gone down, since the risks of contracting these STIs are now much lower because treatments are now so effective. Plus the design hasn't moved along much since the 1950s (more on the future of condoms below).

What is it?

The male condom is a sheath that rolls over the penis and is usually made of latex. The female condom lines the inside of the vaginal canal and are made of a similar material. The effectiveness of the male condom is 98% while the female one is 95%. It's likely that this is because the female condom is a bit harder to use correctly. Sometimes the penis can slide down the outside of the condom rather than going into it. Female condoms aren't very popular. They're big, unsexy and more expensive. They're also harder to get hold of. So let's focus on the male one!

How does it work?

It's a barrier method. This means it stops the sperm from ever coming into contact with an egg. Male condoms are easy to use and you only need to use them during sex. They are also the only way to protect against sexually transmitted infections (STIs).

Potential side-effects

There are no medical side effects to using condoms, aside from maybe discovering you're allergic to latex, for which there are alternative options now: polyurethane and polyisoprene. I'd like to look at some of the downsides to condoms and try to remedy them, as it's so important to use condoms for STI protection.

You may find condoms practically soak up your natural juices, like a flippin' sponge, leaving you feeling dry and chafed. I'd recommend using a natural condom-friendly lubricant as a back up for this scenario, or just change it up and go for "outside sex".

It can interrupt the flow of sex but this can be overcome with practice. Most men have already done the practice in their bedrooms at home and are pros at slipping on a condom in no time. If the condom "fails" (aka breaks or slips off) you should go to a pharmacy, GP or walk-in center (if in the UK). They will be able to give you the morning after pill, or you can get an IUD from a sex clinic or GP (if they provide contraceptives). Although, if you already practice the fertility awareness method you may be confident that you're not within your fertile window and therefore don't require emergency contraception.

A bit of history

We are very pro-crafts nowadays – from macramé plant hangers to Christmas wreaths, we've done it all. But have you ever made your own condom? No? Well in the 1600s people would make them at home using sheep intestines. I don't recommend it.

The famous Casanova wore condoms made of linen in the eighteenth century. When vulcanised rubber was invented in 1838 by Mr Goodyear, of Goodyear tires, the first reusable condom soon followed. As late as the 1950s men could get condoms on prescription to protect them when having premarital or extramarital affairs. But they couldn't request them to protect their wives from unwanted pregnancies! (Brandt, 1985)

This is because they believed wives were for making babies, not sexual pleasure. It was once believed that it was more sinful for a man to ejaculate outside of his wife's vagina than it was for him to rape someone, because at least the rape might end in a baby . . . This belief that sex, without potential conception, is sinful still resonates strongly in the USA where until 2010 $100 million of federal funds were being spent annually on abstinence-only sex education (NIAIAD, 2001).

In the 1960s condoms became unpopular because the pill and IUD provided protection from pregnancy instead. However, when the virus that can cause AIDs was identified the media and government-led advertisements raised the profile and popularity of condoms once more. Sadly, this health awareness doesn't seem to be enough to encourage the youth of today. But with a design that hasn't changed much since the 1950s, what do you expect?

Enter the future of condoms

There has been A LOT of development in materials since the 1950s and this is finally rubbing off (haha!) onto condoms:

Hex by Lelo is a condom that is made of hexagons of material that makes it feel more natural. (The FDA doesn't allow them to say it's more pleasurable, but it probably is!)

Hanx has breathed new life into the design of condoms by making theirs vegan and so sexy to look at you'd want it in your purse even if you were not tryin' to pull.

TheyFit has a remarkable 66 sizes to choose from. That's right; condoms are not a case of one-size-fits-all. 80% of men have smaller penises than the average condom, the average penis length being 5.2 inches and the range being from 1.6 to 10.2 inches (Sarner, 2017).

So don't just settle for boring old Durex; why not try something new and see how it affects your sex experience? Could be fun. Fun and safe. Two things I always look for in a good night out.

THE COPPER COIL

While I've no personal experience with this method, it's the most popular method aside from FAM (The Fertility Awareness Method) among my friends. It's low-maintenance, long lasting and doesn't affect your hormone cycle (although it may affect your periods). In the USA, Planned Parenthood (the leading contraceptives provider there) saw a 900% spike in IUD fittings in the first few weeks of Trump's presidency as women were terrified their right to contraceptives would be taken away from them (Frizzell, 2017).

What is it?

It's a T-shaped bit of plastic that is wrapped in a coil of copper (hence the name "coil"!). It has strings at the bottom of the plastic T that will dangle out of the cervix so that you know it's still in place and it can be more easily removed. You should check they are in place regularly and if they're not there one day, go to the doctor, as it may not be working anymore. It is more than 99% effective, which means about 1 woman in 100 will get pregnant during a year of using an IUD.

How does it work?

The copper on the IUD acts as an antimicrobial that changes the make-up, ph and consistency of your cervical mucous, thereby preventing sperm from surviving very long. The object itself acts as a minor local irritant, preventing the endometrial lining from thickening and therefore fertilised eggs from implanting (if the sperm ever made it past the inhospitable cervical mucous) (Jonsson et.al., 1991). Depending on the brand it will be effective from 5–10 years.

Potential side-effects

The change to the cervical mucous could change your experience of sex. This isn't something I've seen written or ever heard talked about but I find (with 11 years of FAM experience) that change in mucous changes my experience of sex so it seems a sensible leap of logic.

Infection is so rare with installation of the IUD it's hardly worth mentioning but the actual rates were very hard to get hold of and this article reference explains why (Hubacher, 2014). If you experience a temperature, pain in your lower abdomen or smelly discharge after having yours fitted you must go to the doctor.

However, as we learn more about the benefits of healthy gut and vaginal flora I think it's worth considering that the IUD's impact on the microbiome of the vagina could create a predisposition for bacterial vaginosis, candida and possibly cystitis (Elhag et.al. 1988), (Parewijck et.al. 1988). The strings that hang into the vaginal cavity attract bacteria and are able to transport those bacteria into the uterus. Whereas usually there is a coating of cervical mucous between these two places which prevents that.

Less than 1 in a 1000 women has a perforated uterus as a result of the IUD fitting (Gov.uk, 2015).

Changes to your period are normal for 3–6 months after having it fitted. For most women they will go away after that. But for others the changes could last as long as the coil is in. You may get heavier (or lighter) periods, they may get longer (or shorter) and they may get more (or less) painful. Sorry to be so vague but I've heard of all these effects in friends with IUDs and while only the things not in brackets are usually listed as "side effects" it's worth pointing out the opposites as sometimes less painful, or shorter, or lighter periods may be perceived as negative by the user! Bleeding between periods is also possible; if you experience this discuss it with your doctor. It's normally not deemed to be a problem.

The IUD may embed into the uterine wall. This happens in up to 18% of women. But the degree of embedding can vary and often goes unnoticed. Embedding doesn't usually affect the effectiveness of the IUD as a contraceptive (RSNA, 2012).

It may be rejected by the body entirely and pushed out. My understanding is that this is rare. Exactly HOW rare, I still can't find a good research paper on. Your risk increases the younger you are and the worse your period pain is (Zhang et.al. 1992).

A bit of history

For centuries people have been shoving stuff up their vaginas to stop babies from coming out. The intrauterine device takes that one step further by crossing the boundary of the cervix. In the ninth century a Persian physician recommended inserting into the cervix paper, wound together into the shape of a probe, tied with string and smeared with ginger water (Manisoff, 1973).

The initial IUD designs would dangle half in the uterus, half out (in the vaginal cavity) which made it a perfect vehicle for bacteria to traverse from vagina to uterus. In a time where gonorrhoea was rife, and antibiotics were non-existent, this was literally deadly. As with most contraceptives they went through massive development during the nineteenth century when contraception became less taboo.

Following that the IUD went through many incarnations and gained in popularity. However, the IUD took a massive nosedive in popularity during the 70s thanks to a faulty model (The Dalkon Shield) finding its way onto the market. It resulted in many pregnancies, miscarriages (often in the 3rd to 6th month) and infections which sometimes led to death. This probably explains why the baby boomer generation didn't recommend this form of contraceptive to their daughters. At the time the federal government in the USA hardly had any rules to ensure quality of these devices (as is the case now for tampons!) but since then regulations have changed significantly. Between 1976 and 1988 there developed the more modern designs of plastic T-shaped IUDs covered in copper, finishing with the progesterone embedded coil most people use now. This was added because it helped to act as a local relaxant for the womb and stopped it from being expelled quite so often while also preventing embedding of an egg. While medical professionals consider the effects of the progesterone localised I have heard women report a change to their overall hormone cycle as a result. More research needs to be done on this. Although this is seen as the most recent version of an IUD, many women are returning to the copper coil as a non-hormonal option.

FERTILITY AWARENESS METHOD

We've already been over FAM a lot so I'll keep this brief.

What is it?

The fertility awareness method is a way of charting your hormones using your waking body temperature, cervix position and texture, and cervical mucous quality to tell where you are in your cycle. It can be used as contraceptive, but also for conception.

How does it work?

Biological changes happen to the recorded signs and symptoms that tell us when ovulation occurred. If this is recorded and calculated accurately sex can be avoided or a barrier method used to avoid pregnancy. It is up to 99% effective.

Potential side-effects
It doesn't have any because it's non-invasive.

A bit of history
It is thought that a form of trying to assess bodily symptoms to tell if a woman is fertile has existed as long as people have been on earth. But the formalised practise of recording as it is now has only been happening since 1964 (Knight, 2017). Its effectiveness has only improved over the years with increased understanding of how ovulation and pregnancy occur. It gets a lot of bad press because a mathematical method called the rhythm method was confused with it. The rhythm method just counted forward 14 days from your previous period to assume you'd ovulate then. Of course, this isn't the case for most women. So it wasn't very effective. Even now, people think that's what you're doing when you use FAM. It's up to you to let them know where their confusion lies.

DIAPHRAGM AND CAP

What is it?
The diaphragm is a disc of latex that is inserted into the vagina to block the cervix from meeting sperm. The cap does the same thing but has more of a cup shape and a smaller diameter.

How does it work?
It is used with a spermicide gel, ensuring any sperm that reaches it dies very quickly. Interestingly, if you're not in the fertile phase of your cycle sperm can only survive for a matter of minutes, perhaps hours, because the cervical mucous traps the sperm and kills it by being the wrong ph (Knight, 2017). Spermicidal gels ensure that your vagina is an acidic environment whenever it's used. The barrier is left in for more than 6 hours before removing it post-coitus.

The cup of diaphragm is inserted any time before sex, but the spermicide needs to be topped up if it has been inside you more than 3 hours without use. You also need to add more after each time a man ejaculates inside you if you want to have sex more than once whilst wearing it. It is between 92–96% effective with the prescribed spermicide (nhs.com, 2018).

Potential side-effects

The spermicidal gel may have side effects upon the vaginal wall but this is thought to only occur if the contraceptive is used very frequently or incorrectly. The spermicide actually damages the top layer of cells in the vaginal wall allowing HIV to be transmitted more readily when it is misused in this way (Wilkinson, 2002). It's best to talk to your doctor about the details of misuse to understand what exactly qualifies.

The diaphragm and cap may increase cystitis in some users, may cause toxic shock syndrome and you may turn out to be allergic to the latex.

Because spermicides are full of manmade chemicals, some people have tried to use those barriers with a natural spermicide rather than the usual one given on prescription. For instance, Neem oil shows some promise as an alternative but it really does smell horrid and research is slim. But if you are combining this method with a male condom, then you might be willing to experiment with natural spermicides, so long as you are aware that their effectiveness is unknown.

A bit of history

Various barriers to the cervix have been applied since records began. Some of the oldest are records of paper discs applied to the cervix by sex workers in Asia. More famously, Casanova is said to have used the ends of lemons. We know now that lemon juice is indeed a spermicide to some extent, presumably largely down to its acidic nature. In the early twentieth century it was illegal to even educate women about contraceptives. Famously, Margaret Sanger was jailed in 1916 for educating women about the diaphragm. She tried to smuggle diaphragms from Germany into New York, but they were confiscated by customs. She protested this decision in court and in 1936 a judge ruled they could be delivered, thereby opening up new possibilities for freedom of choice in the USA.

In 1941 the diaphragm was the most popular form of contraceptive, but its use nearly completely died out with the invention of the contraceptive pill. By 2002 only 0.01% of the USA population still used it, and yet it was once featured in an episode of Sex in the City when the main character Carrie Bradshaw was to ask her friends for help in retrieving her diaphragm from her vagina after a great night out with a lover.

Wellness   Problem   Illness

*

⟶

If any of the things in this section happen you want to firstly feel assured by your doctor that it isn't being caused by an illness. If it isn't, you can feel comforted that the recipes in the book should be enough to help. This advice is as practical as I could make it.

How stress affects periods

There are many ways your period may change in your lifetime. Sometimes it'll be part of natural ageing, sometimes it'll be a sign of disease, but the rest of the time it gets called "unexplained" and is usually "untreatable". I've been told plenty of times that my symptoms are "normal" and there is nothing to be done.

But I want you to know there is ALWAYS something that can be done – even if it's not a cure, improvements can always be made. This section is so you can be aware of the possible causes of the problem you experience, and can press for tests when you need them.

Getting told by a doctor there is nothing wrong with you when you experience a problem can feel like purgatory. Trapped somewhere between wellness and illness with no way to ensure you get back to wellness. I was lucky to find the tools I needed to do this, tools I'll share in this book. The first step was knowing it was stress that had got me there in the first place.

THE 3 STAGES OF STRESS

The trouble with stress is that most of us haven't a clue about how stressed we are. When I was doing 14 days straight of work, I felt tired, I didn't feel overwhelmed or unable to cope, I certainly didn't identify as stressed, I was on fire! It's only now that I look back, with clearer eyes, I can see that it may not have felt stressful but it was stressful. You can imagine my happiness when I discovered there's a psychological hypothesis that explains it all!

Hans Selye (1907–1982) came up with a model for stress called general adaptation syndrome. This features 3 stages of stress, each of which requires a different herbal treatment protocol. It's common for people to misuse herbs in self-treatment because of this. Let's have a little look at the different stages, and herbs for each.

Stage 1. Alarm reaction

This stage is the one we are most familiar with. This stage is characterised by short bursts of stressful scenarios where the body has the typical flight or fight reaction. Adrenaline levels rise, the heart and breathing rate increases, and focus improves. We evolved this reaction to help us avoid being eaten by things when we were hunter-gatherers. Now we initiate it for a myriad of things, whether it's work, relationships, money problems or emergencies.

This reaction is generally beneficial in the short term as it increases our ability to cope with a stressful scenario. The body should naturally shift into a rest and relaxation mode once it has passed. To help it do this you can use herbs called relaxants. Many herbs fit into this category and we will cover only a few here.*

Chamomile is a herb worth knowing. People that find it doesn't work just haven't had a decent quality version of it. I'd recommend Neal's yard remedies, Baldwins, and Pukka for good teas. Chamomile is a very gentle relaxant suitable for almost anyone. It can help relieve anxiety and tummy upsets, as well as helping you sleep at night.

Lemon balm has a lovely fresh lemon taste and as part of the mint family it grows rampantly once it's decided it likes where it is. You can have it as tea or add a few leaves to cold water in summer for a refreshing drink.

---

* You can look up these herbs in the second part of the book for more details.

Skullcap is a great herb if you're finding your mind keeps going over a scenario. I use it in blends whenever someone can't sleep for thinking too much.

Stage 2. Adjustment

If stress continues the adjustment stage begins. During this stage the body adjusts the output from the adrenals in an attempt to maintain a higher level of productivity for longer. Essentially your body starts to pace itself as though it's in a race. During this stage you may cease to recognise just how stressed you are because you have adjusted to a constant level of it.

At this point it is important to use herbs called adaptogens. This is a group of herbs researched after World War Two to essentially make super soldiers. They were found to minimise the impact of long-term stress on the body and increase longevity. Most of these herbs aren't native to the UK, possibly because the research was done by the Russians, who had easy access to the Chinese pharmacopeia.

These herbs are great if you know you'll be going through something stressful for more than a week, e.g. Exams, moving home, weddings, funerals etc. They are complemented nicely by the relaxants from stage 1.

Rhodiola rosea is a fairly well known herb because it helps minimise stress as well as improve symptoms of depression.

Liquorice root is a sweet adaptogen that helps to soothe the digestive system, especially when it is prone to constipation. However it's not recommended in those with high blood pressure. I always take a stick of liquorice whenever I have an audition or interview to calm my nerves.

Ashwaghanda is an Indian plant coming from the Ayurvedic herbal tradition. It is used to strengthen the adrenals as well as support the immune system. Great if you tend to come down with colds when stressed.

Stage 3. Exhaustion

At this stage the body has run out of its natural energy resources and immunity is extremely low. This is often referred to by herbalists as adrenal exhaustion. You may notice fatigue which you can't shake, anxiety, depression and recurring infections. It's important at this stage to use herbs which help to build the energy reserves back up again. Herbs which do this are often called tonics.

Nettle is a general tonic high in vitamins B,B,C,D, and K as well as iron. It is excellent for balancing immunity as it has natural antihistamine which helps reduce allergic reactions like asthma and hay fever.

Oat straw is a nervous tonic. It helps to coat the nerves and reduce their sensitivity. This makes it good for reducing anxiety and nervousness.

Hawthorn is a cardiovascular tonic. Excellent for balancing both high and low blood pressure by strengthening the entire system. It can help with anxiety, palpitations and sleep troubles alike.

It's important at this stage to use adaptogens from stage 2 but often the relaxants from stage 1 are not so useful. Relaxants for someone who is already exhausted can often create even more tiredness. This is the body's natural way to repair itself so it makes sense. However, someone with fatigue is rarely looking to rest more. This stage is best treated under the supervision of an experienced herbalist. I have seen adaptogens overstimulate very depleted people, worth bearing in mind.

THE PROGESTERONE STEAL

I experienced first hand how stress can affect periods. While mine created an exacerbation of constriction and inflammation, many women experience a change to the regularity and flow of their periods, sometimes stopping altogether. There is an important biological process which links our reproductive system with stress which I'll go into now, but not without a story first.

My husband and I were visiting a grand old house in Wales, on our way to a Christmas getaway. In the house was a dining room, set out as it would have been in the Victorian era. It was a cold and blustery day. Upon this table was a few golden candelabras with nature inspired motifs and golden pineapples.

"Wouldn't it be nice to have some of these decorations for our own Christmas?", my husband remarked. "Why would I want a symbol of white men raping and pillaging foreign lands on my table at Christmas?", I replied.

It was a tad negative, I admit, and when my husband pointed out that, if we were to impose a ban on all fruits from places white men had raped and pillaged from, we would be missing a large portion of our Christmas pudding . . . I soon backed down.

We've all overreacted at some point in our lives. Some are more emotional while others, quite physical. Take, for instance, your inbox at work. I have received emails from my boss marked "urgent" which instantly make my heart race, my breath quicken and my palms sweat. That uncontrollable panic is a little something called the flight or fight response. It was designed for use against the pursuit of lions and yet here we are, using it for digital messages shone at us from a computer screen.

This response is fuelled by a hormone called cortisol and its production has another helpful yet harmful side effect. It can stop you from conceiving. You see, we have this amazing inbuilt protection against babies in times of stress. The body can either ovulate or it can enable the flight or fight response. The more stressed we are, the less FSH and LH the body makes, inhibiting ovulation. Stress also changes how we process insulin, and interferes with all hormone reactions. Some say this is called the "progesterone steal" but this seems to be an oversimplification of how stress changes our hormones.

Previously it was thought there was one pool of pregnenolone, which could either be turned into progesterone OR cortisol, not both. But we now know there are smaller stores of pregnenolone in a variety of endocrine glands all over the body. This makes it hard for the idea that cortisol and progesterone are competing with each other to exist so simply as it is posed in the progesterone steal theory. We have to look higher up in the scheme of things to the hypothalamus, often seen as the master controller of hormone cascades, to explain how stress effects periods (McCulloch, 2018).

Stress tells our hypothalamus to instruct the entire body to respond in a multitude of ways, such as lowering LH and FSH (as mentioned before), for which the end result is less fertility and ovulation. It's how something so simple as an email (or more precisely, a barrage of high-stress emails over a long period of time in a job you absolutely hate) could make you miss a period!

But this isn't the case for all women. Some will have periods but not ovulate, others will have irregular cycles and some might have longer bleeds. For some, it contributes to or causes a condition called Polycystic Ovarian Syndrome (PCOS) where the body has too little progesterone and a relative excess of androgen. It often creates insulin resistance, acne, male hair patterns and sometimes weight problems. So it's important they try to manage their stress as well as their nutrition and blood sugar levels. If you are concerned about stress, and how it may be affecting your cycle, here are my essential tips for improving the situation.

There is a big difference between experiencing the occasional missed period and a condition like PCOS. In my obstetrics and gynaecology textbook it describes what we'll cover in this book as "normal menstruation and its disorders". I couldn't possibly differentiate between short-term stress or an undiagnosed condition from the other side of these pages. That's why, if a period change causes you concern or becomes a pattern, not a one-off, it is imperative to see your health professional. You don't have to take the medicines they offer if you don't want, but in the UK it is the cheapest way to first get a diagnosis. Then you can choose how you want to treat it by investigating all the options; herbal medicine, acupuncture or nutrition being my favourite places to start.

The following chapters will look at different period changes stress could lead to and the conditions they signify. If these changes are addressed and balanced early enough a condition should not occur. If, on the other hand, you're already experiencing a condition, then the tips herein should support you on your journey to wellness, though I don't think they would cure on their own. If they do, email me!

The science of slow living

I experienced terrible period pain and anxiety, but never was I diagnosed as sick. My pain actually was neither severe enough, nor long-lasting enough to be considered that. But it changed my day-to-day life in a negative way nonetheless. That's why I knew there would be countless women told they needed to either put up with it, take painkillers, or stop bleeding (aka take the pill or get pregnant) just like me. When I found remedies which worked for me and understood how important stress management was, I knew I had to share it with the world.

My first lesson in stress was learning about the different sides of the nervous system and what they do. This understanding has become an integral lesson I teach all my patients. Let's try it now as an exercise:

Remember the path:

Wellness   Problem   Illness

Keeping this in mind, turn to the chart on the opposite page. Here, you can note what you do, the time of the day you do it, and, without thinking too much about it, mark it as "active" (A) or "passive" (P) »»

Important — Don't read on until you have done this exercise, even though this means putting the rest of this book on hold for a day or so.

TIME	WHAT I DO	A/P
5–6		
6–7		
7–8		
8–9		
9–10		
10–11		
11–12		
12–13		
13–14		
14–15		
15–16		
16–17		
17–18		
18–19		
19–20		
20–21		
21–22		
22–23		
23–24		

The nervous system is split into two distinct parts; the sympathetic nervous system (we will call this the "active" part) and the para-sympathetic nervous system (which we'll call the "passive" part).

The active part of the nervous system gives us the infamous flight or fight response. In this, the pupils dilate, digestion slows down, the heart beat races and you may lose control of your bladder.

The passive side of the nervous system gives us the less well known rest and relax response. While we are using the passive side our pupils contract, the heartbeat slows, digestion is activated and we have full control of our bladder.

Now, go back, and recategorise each thing you do during the day. Do they seem active or passive now?

You'll begin to realise quite quickly that each thing you do can be approached one way or the other. There are active ways to read an article and passive ways. There is an active way to eat your meal, shoving a sandwich in your gob while rushing to your next meeting, and a passive way, eating your meal at a table with family and sharing your day's tribulations.

Tally up the total actives and passives and see how your day compares. Are you spending more hours in the active state or the passive state? Do you need more passive time in your life? Or more active?

What people don't realise, is that in order to have an efficient flight or fight response we have to spend at least as much, if not more time resting and relaxing. When we are passive (i.e., resting and relaxing) we are repairing our bodies both physically and mentally. When we spend extended periods of time in the active state we end up with colds, then tiredness/insomnia, and finally exhaustion and chronic fatigue. This "story" of extended periods of time spent in "active mode" is the starting point of most of my patient's explanation of how they got sick. It's my job to teach their minds and bodies to use the passive side again, and that's where slow living comes in.

Here are some of my favourite slow living "activities" that help engage the passive side of the nervous system:

» Most crafts such as knitting and crochet
» Most creative outlets such as drawing and singing
» Meditation
» Long baths
» Reading
» Painting your nails (because it stops you doing anything while they dry!)
» Getting a massage or other relaxing treatment
» Turning off the internet on your phone for certain hours of the day (or all alerts if you're a total phone addict like me)
» Taking your lunch AWAY from your desk each day at work
» Having tech-free evenings, (that includes no TV and no internet)

This is a tiny list of things you can do. Each person will have different things that switch on their passive side of the nervous system and it's important that you experiment with different things and remain mindful and attentive to your needs as an individual. The key thing to remember is that you don't actually have to change your daily habits. You just need to change the way you do them. Food is a great opportunity for this. It's far more beneficial to your wellbeing if you take your full lunch break, away from your desk, somewhere peaceful, and eat something healthy or homemade (or both!) as opposed to shoving a sandwich in your mouth at your desk whilst continuing to check emails.

People really take for granted the simple fact that rest allows you to work so much more efficiently. Taking a short break when you're feeling tired can mean that you come back able to complete a task that you had been struggling over for hours in a matter of minutes.

RELAXATION IS A SKILL

When I was working those long stints at Neal's Yard Remedies I was in Stage 2 of stress. Over time though, as I started to slip towards stage 3, I began to experience anxiety and severe fatigue. Each month, I'd feel totally wiped out for one or two days in my premenstrual phase. But by learning how to be passive I was able to rein it back in and recharge my battery again. The first thing I did was take less work.

As it turned out though, the absence of work is not equivalent to relaxation. I've had to learn how to relax and now I think of it as something I do. Not something that happens to me.

Are you working too hard? It can be hard to tell. Not all of us show signs of stress in the same way. It's important to understand that we all have different signs from our bodies but here are some of the most common I see:

> » Unexplained migraines
> » Difficulty falling asleep
> » Difficulty staying asleep
> » Waking up tired
> » Panic attacks and anxiety

» Unexplained menstrual problems, especially heavy or nonexistent periods
» Chronic muscle tension
» Recurring infections

If you have some of the above you need to know what stage of stress you're in to choose the right herbs for the situation. Take the test below to get an idea of where you might be at.

STRESS TEST

How do you feel today?

a) Feeling a bit panicked and wired today
b) I feel fine
c) I've been feeling worried/depressed for a while now

How are you sleeping?

a) I can't get to sleep
b) I have no trouble sleeping
c) I can't stay asleep

What do you crave?

a) I crave chocolates and sweets
b) I can't get by without coffee
c) I'm off my food at the moment

How often do you get sick?

a) Never
b) Once a year
c) All the time!

How are your energy levels?

a) I wake up tired
b) I get a mid-afternoon slump
c) I pass out on the sofa each night

Now tally up which letter you selected most and read the appropriate analysis.

Mostly As

If you answered mostly As you're the best kind of stressed. You can tell that you feel stressed and it comes in waves. This is the sort of stress we were biologically designed to feel. It's famously referred to as the flight or fight response. It gives us the energy to get what needs to be done, done. But it does tend to put us off our food and it can make life tiring when it becomes a pattern. What's important is that you use a class of herbs called relaxants, like chamomile.

Mostly Bs

You're mid-level stressed. You've become so accustomed to being stressed you don't even feel it anymore. But that doesn't mean it's not affecting you. You probably struggle to sleep or feel like you never get enough. You may notice that you are always reaching for sugary treats too. Liquorice is an adaptogen that helps you to rejuvenate when you're going through long-term stress. It increases stamina and nourishes the digestion.

Mostly Cs

I'm afraid you're max-level stressed. This means you've been going through stress for a very long time indeed. It's worn you down and now you need to concentrate on nourishing yourself, taking time to rest and relax. Nettle is like a food. It's high in vitamins A, B, C, D and K as well as iron. It can be drunk as often as you want but you should have it at least 3 times a day.

It's not easy to identify what stage of stress you're in as the tendency is to rationalise how well you're coping instead. This is where a herbalist comes in handy. They can look at things objectively and get the herbs right for what you need. But, as a general rule of thumb, if you feel stressed, take relaxants and if you have symptoms but no stress then take adaptogens.

You will never be "given" the time to relax. Time to relax is something you fight for, every week, to achieve. It's whenever you say no to some extra work. It's when you don't answer a text because you just sat down to dinner. It's when you book a massage on the weekend. It's when you ask a colleague to help you out because you're struggling instead of doing it all yourself.

Relaxation is a skill. Learn it.

How I survived adrenal fatigue

When I was teetering on the edge of exhaustion (stage 3) it was much easier to see my wellbeing was out of whack than when I was a functioning stressaholic. I took serious measures to get myself out of the hole. Not only did I cut back on work but I started to introduce relaxation techniques and speed up the process with medicinal herbs too.

I try not to think of myself as weak, but it's hard not to when your physical capabilities seem so much less than others. Although I have a robust immune system and hardly get sick in that way, it's easy for me to get carried away in a fit of creative passion and work myself into a stupor. The same thing happens if I go out socialising all the time, but faster. I find it hard to be around people because I can't help but wrap my consciousness up in theirs. I spend a lot of time trying to understand people. It's what I do for a living. But I find it hard to switch that off. So if I'm not working late on my latest projects

I'm busy trying to get in someone's head. I have learnt that I need to be careful to spend time alone to mitigate the effects that day to day relating with people has on me.

Some would call me an empath. I love the concept but I don't walk around being constantly invaded by others emotions as may be expected of an empath. I listened to a great podcast, called Invisibilia, which interviewed a lady whom this happens to. She had chosen a life of isolation as a result.

Last Christmas when I worked myself into a state of fatigue I chose the same thing. I actively avoided going out, especially into London. The train, full of noise, people, and lights, was just too much for my senses to handle. More recently I started to notice some of those feelings returning, and I knew I must be run down. During this time I would get totally exhausted in the week before my period, and get terrible period pain which stopped me working for as much as 3 days a month (hardly anything compared with someone who has endometriosis though).

So I took some serious herbal, nutritional and lifestyle measures to get myself back on track again. These remedies won't suit everyone in the same situation. But it's a nice place to start your experiments.

REMEDIES

Liquorice and rehmannia decoction

This beefy remedy is made of two Chinese herbs. The Chinese have amazing methods for preparing their herbs. The rehmannia is fermented before being dried and the liquorice is honey treated before being dried. I'm not completely sure those things happen before its dried actually so don't take my word on it. I work at Middlesex University sometimes in their Park Clinic where the students from different herbal traditions learn their trade. I was smelling and tasting the Chinese herbs one day and felt particularly drawn to these two. I already knew liquorice as an adaptogen, brilliant for stress and recovery from fatigue but didn't know much about rehmannia.

I took some home anyway and decocted it like so:

1. I took about 5g of each and covered with cold water over night in a saucepan.
2. The next day I brought it to boil and simmered for 10 min.
3. I had a little mouthful that day and was so nourished by the taste I put the rest in the fridge.
4. I consumed it, a mouthful each day, from the fridge for the next 5 days or so.

The sweetness and savoury taste of this blend was fantastic and I could tell from how much I enjoyed the strong taste that it was giving me what I needed. I trust my senses when it comes to taking my medicines and take it when I find the taste serves me and no longer than that. Getting to know your body this intently takes years but is well worth it.

Lime blossom deep decoction

Lime blossom (*Tilia*) is a beautiful summer herb with lovely relaxing properties. It helps you unwind and take the burdens of life off your shoulders. When I first tasted this preparation of the herb I felt like I was unfurling, like a coiled up flower, opening for the first time.

1. Take fresh or dried *Tilia* and cover with water until it's happily swooshing about in liquid.
2. Put it in a pan and cover it with a lid.
3. Put the pan in the oven on the lowest heat for four hours.
4. Strain off the liquid and put aside for later.
5. Cover the herb with fresh water and put back in the oven, covered as before, for 8 hours (or overnight).

6. Now strain this new decoction and combine with the first straining.

7. Put this on the hob with a lid on and bring to the boil, then simmer for 12 hours (or until it reduces to half its volume).

I kept my deep decoction in a sterilised glass container in the fridge for weeks and it hasn't changed at all so far, so I think the shelf life will be excellent on it. (I'll soon be interviewing the genius behind this method, Cristina Cromer, for the podcast). I took between 10ml and 30ml of this each day until I forgot about it. I usually take it as a good sign when my patients forget to take their medicine. The problem can't be very troublesome if it doesn't remind you to take your medicine!

LIFESTYLE HABITS

Sleep

The hardest part of sleeping for me is sticking to a routine, and during the summer the long days naturally keep me awake for longer. When the days were at their longest I actually closed the curtains and plunged myself into darkness sooner to trick my pineal gland into thinking it was time for bed. The best thing I ever bought for summer was a blackout shade from the Early Learning Center. The quality of sleep is so much better without the sun waking you up at 4am!!

Delegate

When things are super-busy I am more diligent than normal to have my to-do list in my diary, and when I can't do things I ask for help. The easiest place to ask for help is in the home. When you work for yourself you can't turn to a team of people to get work done for you. But you can, hopefully, ask your partner (or family member) to help you by making sure dinner is on the table and the house isn't a state. I've even hired virtual assistants to help me during my super-busy times. There's only so much one person can do. The sooner you accept that the better.

NUTRITION

Instant meals

When you're tired you eat rubbish and rubbish food makes you tired. Here's my quick-fix-lord-help-me-i-need-some-vitamins-meal.

1. I take miso soup mix from Clear Springs.
2. Throw in some egg noodles, some dried seaweed and soak some medicinal mushrooms.

The saltiness is exactly what I need when I'm low. Hope that helps!

Wellness   Problem   Illness

———————————————————————————————✱——————————

                    ————————————▶

When stress and periods mix
[How we go from well to ill]

HEAVY BLEEDS

Heavy bleeding really sucks. The constant worry of it seeping through your clothes, that weird hot flood of blood when you stand up, the extreme lethargy! Many women end up too scared to leave the house as a result. But how much is too much? I have a medical reference book that says "if periods are reported as unacceptably heavy, then they are"!

I love this definition. No more ambiguous measurements that no one (except menstrual cup users) can actually measure. No more "how many pads do you get through in a day?" Whatever you find unacceptable is too much. End of.

If someone tells me they have to get up in the night numerous times to change their sanitary product, that raises red flags for me. I feel the same if a patient says they wear multiple products at once, e.g. a tampon and a pad or a pad on top of another pad.

The fancy term for heavy periods is *Menorrhagia*. If you are ever diagnosed with this, don't be fooled, it's just the Latin word for heavy periods. It doesn't mean they know anything much about what the cause is. In fact, in 50–60% of women never do find a cause and this gets called dysfunctional uterine bleeding, or DUB for short (Collins et.al., 2013). It's a diagnosis of exclusion. Once they know nothing else is happening you are awarded the DUB prize!

What to do

Firstly, make sure it isn't being caused by any disorders such as the ones below. Once you've had it confirmed to be "normal" for you, you can get on with treating it. If it is caused by a reproductive disorder the most effective way to treat it is to treat that. But, as in many cases, where the menorrhagia is happening with no known reason you can get straight on with taking herbs and supplements to help.

Possible reproductive causes
» Fibroids
» Uterine or endometrial polyps
» Endometriosis
» Adenomyosis
» Pelvic inflammatory disease
» Contraceptives such as the IUD

Other causes
» Abnormal prostaglandin ratios
» Anaemia
» Coagulation defects
» Hypothyroidism
» Liver disorders
» Blood disorders
» Adrenal disorders

Normal life-events as cause
» Menopause
» Pregnancy
» Menarche (first year of periods can be erratic and different from what they will become)

Diagnosis

> » Hysteroscopy (camera in the uterus through the abdomen)
> » Ultrasound

It's worth considering the side effects of these diagnostic techniques. Always do a cost/benefit calculation in your head before going ahead. When I had very bad period pain the first diagnostic skill that would have been most useful would have been a hysteroscopy and biopsy. But, whenever you undergo surgery, scar tissue can be left behind. This could have interfered with my fertility and I was yet to have any children. At that time, it made more sense for me to try treating it without checking for things like endometriosis because I wasn't willing to potentially compromise my fertility. The pain wasn't bad enough for that.

It's important that you make your decisions with all the information available to you. Don't avoid a procedure just because it seems scary. Get the facts. What's the worst-case scenario with the treatment, what's the worst without? What's the actual statistical likelihood of that worst-case scenario occurring? I can't guide you on these decisions. You must speak to someone who can give you all the details on the procedures and the actual statistics (don't settle for "it's unlikely to happen"). At the end of the day, the risk level your doctor is comfortable with may be different to yours!

Emotions

Whenever I see a patient with heavy bleeds they tend to be women who are serial-carers. They give all their energy and time to others. They may expect something in return, but rarely get it. They are literally letting their life blood flow from them.

But I remember, once, I had a patient, who was very good at looking after herself. So she puzzled me. It took a few appointments to realise she had someone in her life that she found draining. Someone she couldn't escape from. Someone she saw every day and who would be so needy she found it hard to function. In this instance, it seemed that rather than her giving energy away, this person was literally sucking it out of her like a vampire.

Normal treatment

- » Ablation
- » Hysterectomy
- » Contraceptive pill
- » Antifibrinolytics (like Tranexamic)
- » Progestogens
- » IUD
- » NSAIDs (like Mefanamic acid to reduce inflammation)

Herbal treatment

- » **Relaxants:** lime blossom (*Tilia cordata*), or rose (*Rosa damascena*). To reduce stress which may lead to a hormone imbalance
- » **Liver support:** marigold (*Calendula officinalis*) or dandelion root (*Taraxacum officinalis rad.*) to clear excess hormones faster
- » **Anti-haemorrhage:** raspberry leaf (*Rubus idaeus*), shepherd's purse (*Capsella*) or lady's mantle (*Alchemilla vulgaris*) to stop heavy blood flow
- » **Phytooestrogens:** marigold (*Calendula officinalis*) to balance oestrogen in the body
- » **Blood tonics:** alfalfa (*Medicago sativa*) and nettle leaf (*Urtica dioica fol.*) to replenish the body after blood loss
- » **Womb tonics:** lady's mantle (*Alchemila vulgaris*) and raspberry leaf (*Rubus idaeus*) to support womb health

Losing blood also means you're losing iron and having less iron means you'll bleed more! So get on with having some iron supplements. Nettle is rich in iron but you may need something stronger like Floradix or Spatone (that are two more different natural options for iron supplement which don't constipate). Vitamin A helps with endometrial growth and Vitamin K for increased blood clotting.

To treat heavy blood flow it's important to consider the many ways this may have occurred. In an average period the blood flow is the result of the endometrial lining sloughing off. The endometrial lining will have begun to grow in response to an oestrogenic surge and continued to grow because of progesterone.

This is why we use phytooestrogens. Don't worry, they don't increase oestrogen, they are actually 10 times less potent than the oestrogen you produce (Trickey, 2003). But what they do is take up the same receptor space and therefore give a little hint of an oestrogenic effect without the full whammy. The oestrogen your body produced can't find a space and ends up being excreted by the liver.

Another technique is to use progestogenic herbs or drugs. These maintain the endometrial lining for longer. Ironically this could make the heavy bleeding worse, but if you have a very short cycle and a heavy bleed, progestogens could be just the thing for you. I'd recommend working with a herbalist before dabbling in progestogenic herbs though, as you could make things worse. This can happen with phytoestrogens but because of the way they work it's far less likely.

Recipes to consider
   » Heavy period protection decoction pg. 149
   » Night time tea pg. 145
   » Adrenal fatigue repair decoction pg. 146

NO BLEED

Don't panic! Unless of course you think you might be unexpectedly pregnant. In which case, panic and pee on a stick!

Once you've ruled out pregnancy as the cause, here are a few things to consider. If it's the first time this has happened don't worry, it's most likely to be just a passing thing, probably caused by stress, travel or illness and it'll come back next month. But even so, there are some steps you can take to try and make sure it doesn't happen again.

What to do

» Chill the fuck out. Book a massage, reduce your commitments, and take relaxing herbs like the ones below.
» Eat some awesome food. Concentrate on low glycaemic index, pescetarian meals for the next month. Avoid refined sugar and carbs.
» Exercise a moderate amount. If you've recently increased your work out routine it could be the cause of your missed period. The body naturally switches off periods during times of extreme exertion to protect it from pregnancy.

If you don't get your period again for another month it's time to visit your doctor who can run blood tests. They will be looking for hormonal imbalances that might be causing the situation. If you don't have a period for 6 months you might get the label "amenorrhea" – it just means lack of periods for 6 months or more.

Possible reproductive causes

» Thyroid imbalance
» PCOS (polycystic ovarian syndrome)
» Unreceptive ovarian syndrome (Collins, 2013)

» Primary amenorrhea (when your period never begins even though puberty has begun)
» Premature ovarian failure
» Hyperprolactinaemia

Other causes
» Obesity
» Underweight BMI
» Excessive exercise (Collins, 2013)

Normal causes
» Pregnancy
» Menopause

The steps I gave to begin with help with these non-hormonal causes; they just might take a while to kick in. If your tests return to say there is no hormonal cause, see a herbalist who can offer personalised advice. There is an introduction to PCOS management later in the book. But for a speedier recovery than these guides can give, see a herbalist.

Diagnosis
» Abdominal ultrasound
» Blood tests for FSH, LH, prolactin levels
» MRI scan of pituitary gland (if hyperprolactinaemia is questioned)

Emotions
When it comes to ovulating we need to be in a place of wellbeing for it to occur. I see a lack of periods as often being a sign that the body feels there are more pressing things to be caring for than conception right now. After all, the body is hard wired to assure we don't get pregnant during times of stress. See the chapter on progesterone steal for more details about this. I

haven't noticed any emotional patterns with this particular problem other than that energy seems to be placed upon external achievements rather than self-care. I can't say that's particularly unique in our society though!

Normal treatment

- » Insulin resistance medication (like Metformin for PCOS)
- » Contraceptive pill
- » HRT (for menopause)
- » Thyroxine (for hypothyroidism)
- » Dopamine agonists (like Dostinex or Parlodel to reduce prolactin)

Herbal treatment

- » **Nutritious tonics:** nettle (*Urtica dioica*), alfalfa (*Medicago sativa*) or raspberry leaf (*Rubus idaeus*) rich in vitamins and minerals to nourish the body
- » **Relaxants:** chamomile (*Chamomilla recutita*), skullcap (*Scutellaria lateriflora*), lemonbalm (*Melissa officinalis*) to reduce stress on a daily basis
- » **Support circulation:** hawthorn (*Crataegus laevigata*), ginger (*Zingiber officinalis*) or cinnamon (*Cinnamomum zeylanicum*) so blood can flow better
- » **Support the liver:** dandelion root (*Taraxacum officinalis rad.*) or yellow dock (*Rumex crispus*) so excess hormones are excreted faster

Recipes to consider

- » Adrenal fatigue recovery decoction pg. 146
- » Anxiety relief tea pg. 148
- » Geranium shea butter melt pg. 151
- » Clary sage and lavender bath salts pg. 152
- » Anti-anxiety hanky insta-comfort pg. 154

» Womb attunement pg. 156
» Circulation stimulant pg. 161
» It's all on me pg. 162

A word of warning on *Vitex*
There is research to show *Vitex agnus castus* will reduce prolactin levels. However, I don't recommend trying it without seeing a herbalist because *Vitex* is so complex. I have seen it make hormonal issues as much as I have seen it relieve things. It's effects are said to be dose dependent, but even after considering the dose carefully I have had patients react in the exact opposite way to which I was hoping! It'll be one of the herbs you hear people rave about, having had miraculously cured them more than most herbs. But it's a risky herb to try because of its propensity to make things worse. You can find your local herbalist on google or send us an email to see one of the team at Forage Botanicals.

LONG CYCLES

If your cycle has been longer than 32 days for 3 months in a row you could have something called oligomenorrhea. It's not a condition, it's just the posh name for having long cycles. It could be totally normal for you but if it's not, it's a good idea to get it investigated. Usually long periods are a sign you're not ovulating (in doctor-speak it's called anovulatory). If you're around 40 or older this is probably happening because you're starting to transition into perimenopause and doesn't require treatment unless it gets uncomfortable for other reasons like hot sweats.

What to do

- » Don't panic. Watch, wait and chart.
- » Keep a record of your cycle lengths, period duration and anything else you're noticing.
- » Eat a low GI diet, exercise in moderation and take the herbs listed below. If it continues for more than 3 months get tests done with your doctor. They will be able to tell a lot from a blood test.
- » If you are diagnosed with PCOS or endometriosis read my intro chapter later in the book. If you get told it's a thyroid thing I'd highly recommend a book called *Your Thyroid*, by Barry Durrant-Peatfield.

For anything else, including being told it's not a hormone problem, see a herbalist. You can always skip the guides and go straight to individualised care with a herbalist for PCOS and thyroid stuff too, of course.

Possible reproductive causes:

- » Polycystic ovarian syndrome (PCOS)
- » Endometriosis
- » Ovarian resistance
- » Hyperprolactinaemia (Collins, 2013)

Other causes

- » Coeliac's
- » Diabetes
- » Thyroid disease

Diagnosis

- » Menstrual history
- » Ultrasound
- » Blood tests
- » Physical exams

Emotions

My patients who have long cycles are usually Type A personalities. They are the go-getters. People who want to get ahead in their professional lives. Most of my patients with PCOS have very busy working lives and don't really know anything other than a high-demand lifestyle. If you've only just started to experience long cycles, or it's a one-off experience, reflect on how the month went before this happened. You may find that it was an unusually full-on working month, or you had a big event to prepare for. Potentially it may be longer because ovulation was delayed by stress, travel or illness. This is a perfectly natural way the body protects against pregnancy. If the problem is short-lived without being caused by a disorder it is likely to pass with the next cycle, but it gives you the opportunity to re-dedicate some regular time to self-care.

Normal treatment
  » The pill (to "regulate" periods)
  » Insulin resistance medication (like Metformin for PCOS)
  » Clomid (to stimulate ovulation as part of fertility treatment)
  » Surgery (in some cases of endometriosis)

Herbal treatment
  » **Relaxants:** passion flower (*Passiflora incarnata*), lime blossom (*Tilia cordata*), or lemon balm (*Melissa incarnata*) to reduce stress levels day to day
  » **Support the liver:** marigold (*Calendula officinalis*) or dandelion root (*Taraxacum officinalis rad.*) to encourage the liver to excrete used hormones faster
  » **Support the endocrine system:** ashwagandha (*Withania somnifera*) or liquorice (*Glycyrrhiza glabra*) to help the body withstand long-term stress

» **Anti-inflammatory:** marshmallow leaf (*Althea officinalis fol.*) or chamomile (*Chamomilla recutita*) to reduce inflammation caused by stress

Recipes to consider
» Night time tea pg. 145
» Adrenal fatigue recovery decoction pg. 146
» Geranium shea butter melt pg. 151
» Clary sage and lavender bath salts pg. 152
» Eliminate pg. 160

SHORT CYCLES

A short cycle can really catch you out. No one wants to feel that rush of warm blood when they're out with no supplies! But cycles have a tendency to shorten and lengthen. It can be quite normal as they adjust to the demands of each month. Mine personally were always within a 3-day range of length. But if you find yourself experiencing a much shorter cycle, that jumps, say, 4 or more days down in length it's worth contemplating why.

What to do

It would be good to learn how to chart your cycle in depth so that you are aware of when you ovulate as well as bleed. You can learn this on my Peaceful Period online course or through books that teach the fertility awareness method. In all likelihood either the first half (follicular phase) or last half (luteal phase) will have shortened. Knowing which gives extremely useful information with regard to which hormone may be struggling a bit.

The cause dramatically changes the hormone-changing herbs you'd use. That's why I haven't recommended any herbs that have a direct impact on the hormones. It's too easy to get it wrong and make things worse!

If you feel concerned about the shortness of your period, or it continues to be short for a few months, you should always see your doctor. They will be able to help with a diagnosis through listening to your experiences and perhaps doing blood tests, a vaginal examination, and/or an ultrasound.

In the meantime, concentrate on eating a wholefood diet of unprocessed foods, and concentrate on adding relaxing habits into your life.

Possible reproductive causes
- » PCOS
- » Uterine polyps
- » Fibroids
- » Asherman's syndrome

Other causes
- » Chronic fatigue syndrome

Diagnosis
- » Ultrasound
- » Blood test
- » Physical examination
- » Hysteroscope

Emotions
I haven't noticed any emotional patterns among people who have short cycles so far.

Normal treatment
Generally not treated unless it continues for a long time. You may be offered the contraceptive pill to "balance" the hormones. This is a misnomer and is covered earlier in the book.

Herbal treatment

- » **Liver support:** dandelion root (*Taraxacum officinalis rad.*), burdock root (*Arctium lappa rad.*), or very strong brew of chamomile tea (*Chamomilla recutita*) to excrete hormones faster and improve nutrient absorption
- » **Tonics:** nettle leaf (*Urtica dioica*), hawthorn (*Crataegus laevigata*) and raspberry (*Rubus idaeus*) to nour-ish the body
- » **Adrenal support:** ashwagandha (*Withania somnifera*) and liquorice (*Glycyrrhiza glabra*) to help abate or repair from the effects of long-term stress

Recipes to consider

- » Eliminate pg. 160
- » Adrenal fatigue recovery decoction pg. 146

IRREGULAR CYCLES

Irregular cycles can make life a terrible mess to organise. Never knowing if you're coming or going, it can be hard for some with painful periods to plan social events. It especially makes it difficult to differentiate between a tired or irritable day from a premenstrual day.

What to do

Firstly consider the natural causes of changes to a period; men-opause and breastfeeding. These both affect the length of a period, one with the eventual return of regular periods, the other with the eventual cessation of them. You can rule those out pretty quickly if you're less than 40 years old and don't have a child attached to your boob most of the time!

Other common and natural causes of irregularity are stress and being underweight. These are by far more common than the illnesses listed opposite.

Start by keeping a record. Everyone should be keeping a record of when they have each period. Memories can be quite deceptive, especially for monthly occurrences. I can barely remember what happened yesterday, let alone a month ago! If you have a record of your irregularity take this to the doctor to help them start investigations.

Possible hormone causes
   » Fibroids
   » PCOS
   » Premature ovarian failure
   » Endometriosis
   » Uterine polyps

Other causes
   » IBS
   » Coeliac disease
   » Ehlers-Danlos Syndromes
   » Thyroid disorders such as systemic lupus, erythrasma, (and other autoimmune conditions)
   » Chronic fatigue syndrome
   » Having an IUD

Normal causes
   » Pregnancy or breastfeeding
   » Stress
   » Overexercise

Diagnosis
   » Ultrasound
   » Blood tests
   » Laparoscopy (for endometriosis specifically)

Emotions

» I haven't noticed any emotional patterns among people who have irregular cycles so far.

Normal treatment

» The contraceptive pill
» Thyroxine (for hypothyroidism)
» Anti-inflammatories (for Coeliac disease)
» Steroids (for Coeliac disease)
» Surgery (in some cases of endometriosis)
» Insulin resistance medication (like metformin for PCOS)

Herbal treatment

» **Relaxants:** chamomile (*Chamomilla recutita*), lime blossom (*Tilia cordata*), or passion flower (*Passiflora incarnata*) to reduce daily stress
» **Anti-inflammatory:** marshmallow leaf (*Althea officinalis fol.*) or chamomile (*Chamomilla recutita*) to relieve inflammatory effects of stress
» **Support the endocrine system:** ashwagandha (*Withania somnifera*) for long-term stress management, and adrenal fatigue
» **Tonics:** nettle (*Urtica dioica fol.*), alfalfa (*Medicago sativa*) or hawthorn (*Crataegus laevigata*) to nourish the body

Recipes to consider

» Night time tea pg. 145
» Adrenal fatigue recovery decoction pg. 146
» Anti-anxiety hanky insta-comfort pg. 154
» Womb attunement pg. 156
» It's all on me pg. 162

LIGHT PERIODS

It's pretty rare that someone complains about light periods but they can be just as worrying as the rest, especially if you're trying to conceive.

What to do

If you have just one light period it's likely to just be a blip, but if it happens the following month or causes you alarm go see your doctor. There isn't anything that can be done at the time of the light bleed to improve it, as they're the result of the last month's hormone levels.

Firstly consider your age as the perimenopause can create lighter periods as they peter out. Then consider your weight because you need to be a healthy weight to create a healthy endometrial lining and period. Periods can stop altogether when you're underweight. Smoking is another potential reason periods get lighter. Probably the most common reason, though, is stress. You can read more about that in the progesterone steal section. If you feel concerned you should visit your doctor to rule out any of the above issues.

A period comes because you a) ovulated and released luteniesing hormone from the hypothalamus and then b) maintained an endometrial lining with progesterone. Either low oestrogen, progesterone or lutenising hormone may be the cause. You'd need to have blood tests to isolate which one it is. There are herbs that can support each issue but I have concentrated on stress as the cause below because incorrect diagnosis can lead to a worsening of the problem.

Possible hormone causes

> » IUD
> » Asherman's syndrome
> » PCOS

Other causes
- » IBS
- » NSAID's
- » Antidepressants
- » Thyroid medicine and thyroid disease
- » Eating disorders
- » Chronic fatigue syndrome

Diagnosis
- » Ultrasound
- » Blood tests
- » Hysteroscope

Emotions

Light bleeds often go hand in hand with people who struggle to nourish themselves, either through a lack of self-love and respect, or just through unfortunate circumstance which steals all their attention elsewhere. I see it most in people who have suffered trauma in their past or those who undereat. The self-critical teens are those I've seen most with this issue. That certainly doesn't mean that you're likely to be this way, it's just what I've seen in my practice.

Normal treatment
- » The contraceptive pill
- » Removal of IUD
- » Insulin resistance medication (like metformin for PCOS)

Herbal treatment
- » **Relaxants:** chamomile (*Chamomilla recutita*), lime blossom (*Tilia cordata*), or passion flower (*Passiflora incarnata*) to relieve daily stress
- » **Blood tonics:** nettle (*Urtica dioica fol.*) and alfalfa

(*Medicago sativa*) to build up blood levels through nourishment
- » **Support the endocrine system:** ashwagandha (*Withania somnifera*) for long-term stress
- » **Phytoestrogens:** marigold (*Calendula officinalis*) to balance oestrogen levels
- » **Circulation stimulants:** ginger (*Zingiber officinalis*) or rosemary (*Rosmarianus officinalis*) to boost circulation and warm the body

Recipes to consider
- » Night time tea pg. 145
- » Heavy period protection decoction pg. 149
- » Womb attunement pg. 156
- » Circulation stimulant pg. 161
- » It's all on me pg. 162

MID-CYCLE BLEEDS

These are usually very light and easy to ignore –but don't.

What to do

Don't ignore it. Go straight to the doctor to get it checked out even if it's just a little bit of blood. It can be a normal side effect of a minor issue or it could be an indicator of cancer. So it should be taken seriously. Reassure yourself that the faster you get it checked the less serious it's likely to be! Sorry to scare you with the C word but I believe in informed decisions, not withholding facts for fear of scaring you.

Possible hormone causes
- » Dysfunctional uterine bleeding (DUB)
- » Endometrial hyperplasia
- » Uterine cancer

» Polyps
» Abnormalities of the cervix
» Ovarian cysts
» Hormonal contraceptives (e.g. the pill or depo-provera injection)

Other causes
Malnutrition and low BMI

Normal causes
» Ovulation
» Pregnancy

Diagnosis
» The diagnosis of DUB is made by excluding the others
» Ultrasound
» Physical exam

Emotions
I've never had a patient with mid-cycle bleeding so have no observations of a "type" of person that tends to have this issue.

Normal treatment
» The contraceptive pill
» Progestogen releasing
» IUD
» Progestogens
» D+C (dilation and curettage where the cervix is dilated and the surface layer of the womb is scraped off)

Herbal treatment
If your mid-cycle bleeding is diagnosed as a hormonal disorder then you should seek treatment for that from a herbalist, or whatever therapist you prefer. If however, it is

deemed as "normal" (aka caused by DUB or your natural ovulation), then you can follow the advice below:

» **Relaxants:** chamomile (*Chamomilla recutita*), lime blossom (*Tilia cordata*), or passion flower (*Passiflora incarnata*) to ease daily stress
» **Blood tonics:** nettle (*Urtica dioica fol.*) and alfalfa (*Medicago sativa*) to build up blood quality. Support the endocrine system: ashwagandha (*Withania somnifera*) to manage long-term stress
» **Womb tonics:** lady's mantle (*Alchemilla vulgaris*), raspberry leaf (*Rubus idaeus*) to improve overall health of the womb

Recipes to consider
» Night time tea pg. 145
» Adrenal fatigue recovery decoction pg. 146
» Heavy period protection decoction pg. 149
» Womb attunement pg. 156
» It's all on me pg. 162

PMS

Over history, there have been many explanations for the "monthly malady" that is currently called PMS. But to this day it remains a biological mystery why us women are "plagued" with premenstrual tension. No one knows exactly what hormone is to blame. Some have theorised progesterone, others oestrogen. It seemed at one point that a quick rise in oestrogen seemed to be the issue for a portion of women. Although oestrogen therapy worked for these ladies they didn't make up the majority.

Turns out, it's not one single hormone and it has never been repeatedly treated by an individual hormonal treatment either. Some treatments in the past have included leeches on the cervix, daily vaginal "massage" from your doctor, electro-cution, being slapped 'round the face with a wet towel and isolation (Laws et.al., 1985).

PMS has been observed in every culture studied around the world and even the mayo clinic says as much as 3 out of 4 women "suffer" with it. In fact, it's so common among women it's difficult to put together a control group for a study of non PMS-ing women to PMS-ing women as they're so hard to come by!

Most women in the UK don't see PMS as a disease, despite a long history of it being treated as such by the medical profes-sion. Pierre Systeme in 1775 described it thus:

> "Sacrificing her health for the procreation of the species, woman throughout her reproductive years was condemned to suffer a monthly indisposition, a condition which approaches, more or less, a state of disease" (Systeme, 1775).

Since being coined as a medical syndrome in the 1950s we have viewed ourselves as afflicted with it.

But there is a massive difference between a syndrome and a disease. A syndrome is merely a collection of symptoms given a name by the medical profession. Whereas a disease is a disorder of the function of the body. But women continue to view them-selves as "afflicted" with said syndrome. Even though it's not a disease. I would argue that by having given it a medical defini-tion we have identified with it as though it were an illness. Something not of ourselves, which is screwing with us, and therefore requires medical intervention. Defining PMS as a syndrome also allows us to suppress emotions like irritation and rage that were, for a long time, considered unfeminine.

Before the twentieth century there were no first hand accounts from women as to their experience of PMS. Till then, all written accounts came from men observing it from their perspective. Is it any wonder we see it so negatively when it was defined by people who have never experienced it for themselves? But PMS shouldn't have to be deemed a syndrome to be recognised and respected.

We have gone so far now as to say it is sexist for men to deny the existence of PMS. But I would argue against it. I think we need to stop seeing it as an affliction. We need to understand that it is so common among women it should be considered normal. It's time we realised that PMT should stand for Premenstrual Truth.

A time when our hormones magnify whatever stress we have been dealing with each month. All too often we brush these feelings off as though they were simply momentary lapses of madness. But, surprise surprise, you get the same lapse of madness the following month. Because in the end, it won't be resolved until you find a way of processing whatever it is that's winding you up.

So where does that stress come from? It is my belief that it is largely environmental in the western world. We live in a society in which we wear our long working hours, lack of sleep and coffee requirements as badges of honour: the honour of who's most tired and wired. Taking time to rest is a rebellious act.

You will achieve a level of productivity, creativity and intuition far greater than you ever could on 4 hours sleep and gallons of coffee. But rest isn't something that happens in the absence of stress. It's something that requires planning and preparation too.

What to do

Don't ignore it. It isn't just something to brush off as being caused by your "bloody womb". Take time to redefine and conceptualise PMS into a magnifying glass for your life – what observations are to be made? It may be worth keeping a record of what pisses you off or upsets you during this time for consideration during your pre-ovulatory phase.

Rather than asking yourself if you have PMS it may be more productive to ask yourself, "why have the changes I go through each month become intolerable to me?". They may have physically got more pronounced but don't assume it's because your hormones are what's changed – look outside of that first. If there is a change to your periods at the same time I would go to a doctor to get any actual illness/disorder ruled out too.

Causes

In my opinion, it is caused by external stimuli being highlighted by normal monthly hormonal changes.

Diagnosis

PMS is simply the medical term for the natural premenstrual phase of the cycle. If symptoms experienced during this phase become a nuisance then it's worth using the natural remedies in this book to alleviate them. Your hormones don't necessarily need changing in any way to deal with the problem.

At the moment you can diagnose yourself by simply running through this list of symptoms. But I believe diagnoses should be reserved for illness, and PMS is not an illness. This list of symptoms is here just to remind you how ridiculous the current definition of this natural phase is.

Symptoms of PMS

Breast soreness	Headaches
Tiredness	Spotty or greasy skin
Weight gain	Changes in sex drive
Acne	Muscle pain
Food cravings	Bloating
Mood swings	Swelling

| Feeling upset | Difficulty concentrating |
| Anxiety | Irritability |

These changes are generally perfectly normal but should be viewed as opportunities to improve your wellbeing. Whilst they are rarely signs of illness they shouldn't be igored. They are letting you know it's time to do some more self-care and live a healthier life. The symptom gives you more clues as to what changes should be made. I can't get more specific here.

Emotions

The emotions experienced during PMS change for each woman. Sometimes it is anger, sometimes tearfulness and for others an increase in anxiety or depression. Keep a careful record of your experience so you can reflect on it during the other phases of your cycle. Whatever external stimuli is creating these feelings shouldn't be ignored. It really does bother you, but probably not as much as the premenstrual phase makes out. However, now that it has been highlighted you have the opportunity to deal with it. This may be through having an honest conversation with someone, it may be that you need to change your work/life balance, or other lifestyle changes. It is so individual I can't generalise.

Normal treatment
- » The pill
- » Antidepressants

Herbal treatment

It's hard to make generalities about PMS as it's individual to the menstruators. But one thing that is guaranteed to make it worse is stress. I am ten times more likely to bite off my husband's head over something small like the toothpaste top being left off, than if I'm feeling chilled.

- » **Relaxants:** Chamomile (*Chamomilla recutita*), lime blossom (*Tilia cordata*), or passion flower (*Passiflora incarnata*) for day to day stress
- » **Adaptogens:** nettle seed (*Urtica dioica fol.*), aswagandha (*Withania somnifera*) for long-term stress
- » **Nervines:** oat tops (*Avena sativa*) to protect the nerves and reduce their excitability

Recipes to consider
- » Night time tea pg. 145
- » Adrenal fatigue recovery decoction pg. 146
- » Geranium shea butter melt pg. 151
- » Anti-anxiety hanky insta-comfort pg. 154
- » Uplift my mood pg. 159
- » Womb attunement pg. 156
- » It's all on me pg. 162
- » Let it out pg. 163

PMDD

PMDD is the ugly sister of PMS. It stands for Premenstrual Dysphoric Disorder and affects 3–8% of ovulaters (Halbriech, U. 2003). It is PMS so severe that your life is impacted every month during the week or two before you start your period. There can be physical and emotional symptoms including suicidal thoughts. We don't yet know what causes it, but if it's anything like PMS it won't be down to a singular hormonal imbalance.

What to do

If you feel an affinity for the description above don't ignore it just because it's a "once-a-month" thing. Seek out help! Talk to your healthcare practitioner, acupuncturist, therapist, herbalist and / or therapist. Don't suffer in silence – this shit is REAL and there are ways to help minimise the symptoms.

Causes

I'd hypothesise that hormones don't cause PMDD, but rather an already depressed, melancholic or manic person is being worsened by their natural hormone changes. In which case it isn't the hormones that will need support but the person as a whole with their mental state.

Diagnosis

PMDD is a relatively new diagnosis. It is diagnosed through a health history taken by the GP and matching your situation with the symptoms below. PMDD was first added to the list of depressive disorders in the Diagnostic and Statistical Manual of Mental Disorders in 2013.

Here are some of the symptoms

Markedly depressed mood

Marked affective lability (that's mood swings to us mere mortals)

Decreased interest in usual activities

Lethargy, easily fatigued

Needing more sleep or getting less sleep

Other physical symptoms like breast tenderness, headaches, joint or muscle pain, a sense of bloating or weight gain.
(Collins, S. 2013)

Marked anxiety

Persistent and marked anger or irritability

Subjective sense of having difficulty in concentrating

Marked change in appetite

Subjective sense being overwhelmed or out of control

What's good about PMDD as an illness is that the symptom list is much more specific than PMS which includes almost everything under the sun. That makes it easier to diagnose a small section of society with it, rather than it being so common it may not be considered an illness.

Normal treatment
- » Antidepressants such as SSRI's
- » Antipsychotics
- » Cognitive behavioural therapy
- » Counselling

Herbal treatment
- » **Adaptogens:** rhodiola (*Rhodiola rosea*), or ashwagandha (*Withania somnifera*) for long-term stress
- » **Nervines:** oat tops (*Avena sativa*) to protect the nerves and reduce their excitability
- » **Antidepressants:** lemonbalm (*Melissa officinalis*), or rosemary (*Rosmarianus officinalis*) to lift the spirits

Recipes to consider
- » Adrenal fatigue recovery decoction pg. 146
- » Geranium shea butter melt pg. 151
- » Antidepressant pulse point pg. 153
- » Uplift my mood pg. 159
- » Womb attunement pg. 156
- » Let it out pg. 163

MENSTRUAL PAIN

Some have said that the period is the tears of a vagina that didn't conceive. I disagree. I don't feel that a period is necessarily a sad thing. I'm sure many of you have been elated at the sight of it, the infamous thank-fuck-im-not-pregnant period. Not all women want to get pregnant. But certainly for some the pain they feel is only sharpened by the emotional sense of disappointment that they did not conceive. It seems that in some cases the physical pain is a manifestation of the subconscious emotional pain they have buried deep. But everyone is different.

What to do

Period pain, without any underlying cause, is called primary dysmenorrhea and affects 90% of menstruating women (Irani, 2018). Of that, 40% need to take medication and time off work to deal with it. I fit into that 40% (Irani, 2018). If you're not sure you have primary dysmenorrhea, then go and see your doctor. Please do your research on the possible side effects of all treatments and tests offered before deciding what you want to do. Over the many years that I've had period pain, I've also been a herbalist. I'm always on the look out for natural answers. Sadly I have not found that one thing that makes the pain go away completely, but I have found a lot that makes it better. But first, why do we get period pain?

Reproductive causes
- » Endometriosis
- » Fibroids
- » Ovarian cysts

Normal causes
- » Dysfunctional uterine bleeding (DUB)

"Normal" period pain (DUB) is caused by contractions of the uterus in response to prostaglandins. Prostaglandins are chemical messengers, which trigger the contractions and help the endometrial tissue break away from the uterus and be pushed out of the body. It's the same as what happens during birth, just with none of the oxytocin pain killing benefits that childbirth has. That's why some women who have experienced severe period pain find childbirth a doddle. It seems to me like period pain is part and parcel of a healthy and effective period. But I don't think it has to be incapacitating.

Diagnosis
- » Internal examination
- » Ultrasound
- » Laparoscopy
- » Blood tests

Normal treatment
- » Anti-inflammatories (such as mefanamic acid)
- » Pain killers (such as paracetomol and codeine)
- » The contraceptive pill
- » Hysterectomy (in extreme cases)

Herbal treatment
- » **Muscle relaxants:** crampbark (*Viburnum opulus*) and chamomile (*Chamomilla recutita*) for cramping muscles
- » **Antispasmodics:** feverfew (*Tanacetum parthenium*) to relieve spasm in muscles
- » **Antiinflammatories:** white willow bark (*Salix alba*), or meadowsweet (*Filipendula ulmaria*) to reduce prostaglandins and other inflammatory processes

Other remedies
- » A hot water bottle is the traditional method to relieve period pains as it helps to relax the muscle tension surrounding it. But you can now get these awesome disposable heat pads, which are so thin you can stick them to your body and wear them under your clothes without anyone knowing.

- » Orgasm is a powerful pain killer as it unleashes

endorphins into the system which are even more powerful than the most powerful opiate drugs. You don't have to make this a particularly romantic experience as you're already in pain. Just use your favourite vibrator.

» Evening primrose oil/fish oils are anti-inflammatory and prostaglandins are inflammatory. The more prostaglandins you have the more painful your period pain will be. Take either of these oils every day during that time of the month.

» Avoid refined sugar because it's inflammatory and encourages prostaglandins. Consider just how much sugar you're having and give it a go. I'd recommend the 8-Week Sugar Detox by Sarah Wilson.

» Drink relaxing painkilling teas like cramp bark, chamomile, lemon balm, or lady's mantle every day throughout your cycle. Then top up with "stat" doses of cramp bark tincture throughout the day if you need to. I usually have 20ml as often as I need it for up to 5 doses within the day. If that doesn't work, I might as well take paracetamol!

» Preliminary trials have shown that magnesium may help with period pain. It is best absorbed through the skin so hot baths with Epsom salts (magnesium rich) or sprays of magnesium are great for lessening the pain.

» Take time to yourself. Giving yourself a day to be quiet when you're due on or in the first day of your period can make a massive difference to your experience of it. A lot of the tension I had during my period could be relieved, and the pain with it, if I was able to sit indoors with a movie, hot water bottle, cup of tea, and absolutely no interaction with real life people. I realise this is a luxury for most, but if you can take the time out, your body will love you for it!

Recipes to consider

» Cramp massage oil pg. 155
» Period cramp relief pg. 164
» Night time tea pg. 145
» Womb attunement pg. 156

OTHER COMPLAINTS

Menstrual migraine

Migraines are like headaches, but are usually more severe and accompanied by tunnel vision, an aura, light sensitivity, nausea or vomiting. If your migraines happen in a cyclical fashion (usually premenstrually or during the period) then you might have menstrual migraines. They are usually exacerbated by the dip in oestrogen that occurs premenstrually, leading to increased prostaglandins and more constriction in the blood vessels. But the hormones are rarely to blame, it's usually stress levels and diet. Try to relax the muscles, balance blood sugar and avoid triggering foods.

Foods

» Eat essential fatty acids
» Avoid dairy, caffeine and alcohol
» Eat low GI foods like brown rice

Habits

» Epsom salt baths
» Shavasana
» Time in the dark

Herbs
> » Lavender (*Lavandula angustifolia*), peppermint (*Mentha piperita*), feverfew (*Tanacetum parthenium*)

Weight change

A change in weight due to water retention is quite natural with the average hormone cycle. But, for some, it's quite bothersome, while for others you'd never even know it was happening. You may notice your feet swell, your rings seem tight or you might feel heavy and bloated. It is a misnomer to think your hormones need balancing as it may not be caused by too much of a hormone but rather a sensitivity to perfectly average levels of said hormone. I'm not sure how you'd find out which situation you were in without having your hormone levels tested. If these simple remedies don't help within a month, find your local herbalist.

Food
> » Eat cucumbers, whole grains, cinnamon

Herbs
> » Nettle (*Utica dioica*), burdock (*Arctium lappa rad.*), cleavers (*Galium aperine*)

Ovulation pains

Ovulation pain (*mittelschmerz*) is felt by approximately 50% of women at some point in their life (Knight, 2017). It's normally felt on one side or the other of the abdomen just above the pelvic bone. We are still unsure as to what causes it, but a few theories exist. Some think it may be the follicle putting pressure on surrounding structures, others think it may be because of peritoneal irritation from blood and fluid or the ruptured follicle, and still others believe it could be from peristaltic contractions of the fallopian tube. Naturally you might think that this sensation tells you exactly when you're ovulating, but sadly it is not a very precise marker of when it occurred as it can happen before, during and even after the event itself (Knight, 2017). Because the cause isn't understood it's hard to recommend remedies for it. I'd recommend concentrating on the cramp relieving tincture in part two of the book and use heat pads to help as well.

Acne

A few spots on the chin or along the jawline, which come and go once a month is how I'd define hormonal acne for the sake of this helpsheet. The spots occur most frequently during the premenstrual phase, but can be during ovulation too. It is caused when the liver struggles to process all the circulating hormones in the body. It is usually a sign that your diet needs improving, as the body should be able to deal with the natural hormone change without spots. But there are many reasons for spots. You must seek advice if the spots cover the entire face, if the spots are accompanied by other symptoms or this advice doesn't work within 2 cycles.

Food
» Avoid refined sugar

Habits
» Face masks

Herbs
» Red clover (*Trifolium pratense*), dandelion root (*Taraxacum officinalis rad.*), burdock root (*Arctium lappa rad.*)

Fatigue/poor sleep

Feeling tired during the day, falling asleep in front of the TV before bed, craving coffee, tea, energy drinks or sugary snacks to keep your energy up are common symptoms of fatigue. If you have trouble getting to sleep you may find the suggestions here helpful, especially if it only comes up once a month. If however, you have trouble staying asleep it's more likely this is a long-term problem for you and you'll need more than what's recommended here. Moreover, if the problem has been going on for months on end and seems to be throughout the cycle I would recommend seeing a herbalist who can get to the bottom of things.

Food
» Avoid refined sugar
» Balance insulin with low GI

Habits
» Relax in the bath, good sleep routine, pamper yourself

Herbs
» Passionflower (*Passiflora incarnata*), skullcap (*Scutellaria lateriflora*), chamomile (*Chamomilla recutita*)

Sore breasts

Accidentally brushing past a stranger can be extremely painful for some women once a month. Breasts can swell and become very sore to touch. It generally happens when oestrogen levels spike in the ovulatory phase but can happen elsewhere. It's rarely a sign of an illness but if it's particularly bothersome or accompanied by changes to your period then you should go get it checked out.

Food
» Avoid refined sugar and foods which are packaged in plastic

Habits
» Try a cold cabbage leaf in your bra

Herbs

» Marigold (*Calendula officinalis*), cleavers (*Galium aperine*), dandelion leaf (*Taraxacum officinalis fol.*)

THE MENTAL BACKLASH

We have all seen how the hormones can affect our moods and mental state. Sadly we still live in the shadow of the term "hysteria", which can often make it hard to really own these emotions, especially when they come along only once a month. Most women I come across explain that their period often takes them by surprise, and it's only once it begins that they realise they need to go back to family members and apologise for the last weeks temper tantrums and tearful outbursts.

But why do we think we need to apologise at all? Sure enough, we shouldn't have been mean but saying "sorry I was about to get my period" is NOT an excuse. We need to learn to recognise these monthly emotions as a part of ourselves. They are not a monthly affliction of the brain. A moment of madness caused by our fluxes. In fact, I think we only strengthen the concept of hysteria when we do excuse our emotions in this way. We end up internalising the sexist term.

We need to start being able to accept our emotions as they are. If you become depressed or anxious at the same time each month it's not because of your hormones; it's a combination of how you're really feeling *along* with a change in hormones.

For some women, depression always happens when their energy levels drop and they start to look inwards, as is what happens during the premenstrual phase; for others, it may happen when they're ovulating because they need more time to themselves than they're getting, and the burst of energy of ovulation is all too much for them.

Sadly, reproductive health problems are very difficult for us to talk about in most societies, and this inability to share can lead to terrible mental health problems. There seems to be so little discussion around mental health and even less around the effects of taboo subjects like miscarriage, infertility, and period pain *on* mental health. Many women hide these problems from their employers, explaining the symptoms away with lies instead. Some women are told to keep their miscarriages secret even from their own families. But why is this the case when things like miscarriages are so common?

It's as though we want to hide the sadness and dark times in our lives. As though society can't handle it. We need to keep talking though and break the menstrual and mental health taboos.

Depression

What to do

Whether your period is causing your depression or your depression is throwing out your period, it's important to get help. I think talking therapies are really important in mental health because it's always good to have some kind of sounding board for your own thoughts. It just helps you put things in perspective. I don't always recommend counselling as it can sometimes drag up the past, but I'd say finding the right counsellor is the crucial thing. I have also found that talking to herbalists and homeopaths also helps. It tends to be more of an active discussion with them, rather than a monologue on your part.

Causes

- » Life events
- » Inherited
- » Poor diet
- » Poor sleep
- » Shift work
- » Seasonal affective disease
- » Thyroid problems
- » Addiction

» Loneliness
» Head injuries

If you're having suicidal thoughts, don't hesitate to call the Samaritans in the UK on: **116 123**.

The tough thing for my depression is that I often don't realise I have it till after it's been and gone. In the past my depression has actually expressed itself as social anxiety (which was mega-confusing). The thought of going out and socialising, or even going to busy places with lots of strangers (e.g., London) was all a bit much for me. My life circumstances have now changed and that has all passed, but not without a fair bit of a fight.

Diagnosis
» Urine test
» Blood test
» Health history – to rule out diseases which could be the cause. Otherwise depression is diagnosed following a consultation with a GP

Normal treatment
» Antidepressants
» Cognitive behavioural therapy
» Interpersonal therapy
» Psychodynamic psychotherapy
» Counseling

Herbal treatment
The most common, dare I say famous even, herb for depression has got to be St. John's Wort. As with most herbs, it got a bit of scientific evidence behind it and the world went mad for it. But sadly it interacts with around 50% of all prescribed drugs. Frankly, it's not worth the risk of taking it alongside any

medication, just in case. (Unless you're seeing a herbalist or doctor who can advise you on this.)

Don't forget, the contraceptive pill is included in the list of things you can't have St. John's Wort (SJW) with.

So let's have a look at some of the antidepressing herbs that are often overlooked thanks to ol' SJW.

» **Lemon Balm.** The antidepressing qualities of this plant come from its wonderful uplifting essential oils. Not that that's the only part of it, but it's something worth noting because the way you prepare and preserve those oils can really change the effects of this herb (Taiwo et.al. 2012).

» **Orange blossom.** This is another herb that has a strong scent. But while lemon balm is, well, lemony, orange blossom is very sweet. I would add a half-teaspoon of this to other tea blends you have of relaxants.

» **Rose.** Rose is for grief. It comforts the lonely or broken hearted. The definition of hygge in a cup in my opinion. You can have a teaspoon of this straight in your tea. But I'd really recommend buying some rose water (distilled) and adding this to your chai, hot chocolate or ashwagandha milk.

Anxiety

What to do

It's so important to share your feelings when you are anxious. Talk to a friend, family member or a counsellor. Don't keep it a secret, there is nothing to be ashamed of. Consider your overall well-being. Sleep and food should be improved first and foremost. Once you've got those down add on a bit of exercise to raise the heart rate each week too. But at the same time you may want to visit your doctor, just to be sure there isn't an illness causing the problem.

Causes
- » Thyroid conditions
- » Heart conditions
- » IBS
- » Endometriosis
- » Chronic fatigue syndrome
- » Life events
- » Adrenal fatigue
- » Shift work

Diagnosis
- » Health history
- » Blood test
- » Urine test

Like depression, your doctor may want to rule out other causes before diagnosing it as anxiety syndrome.

Normal treatment
- » Cognitive behavioural therapy
- » Beta blockers
- » Antidepressants
- » Anticonvulsants (such as pregabalin)
- » Sedatives (such as benzodiazepines)
- » Counselling

Herbal treatment
- » **Relaxants:** chamomile (*Chamomilla recutita*), lime blossom (*Tilia cordata*), or passion flower (*Passiflora incarnata*) for day to day stress

» **Adaptogens:** nettle seed (*Urtica dioica fol.*), ashwagandha (Withania somnifera) for long-term stress

» **Nervines:** oat tops (*Avena sativa*) to protect the nerves and reduce their excitability

Even if you don't want to take medicine from a doctor I'd highly recommend going just so they can help give you a diagnosis. Herbalists are also qualified to make this judgement. Without it, you will find it very hard to know what exactly the problem is that you need to treat. This book is mostly written for people who, after all this, were told "nothing" is causing the problem and therefore no treatment is available. The herbs recommended are safe and suitable for everyone. There just may be the occasional situation where an individual just doesn't suit the herb.

What to do in a doctors appointment

» Bring your records of what you've been experiencing.

» Give as much detail, in a chronological order, as succinctly as possible (quite the art form).

» Ask what the doctor would recommend.

» If they don't mention the tests you already had in mind, ask if they think it would be appropriate.

» Because appointments are so short in the UK you must remember that this can be a long process as each part of the journey to a diagnosis is in tiny bite sized pieces, put in order or priority by your doctor.

» If you find yourself bumping heads with your doctor then just book in to see a different one as soon as possible and see where you get with that. If that doesn't work, then, I'm afraid, you'll probably have to go private. It can be worth doing so to get tests faster, which you can then return with the results to your GP who can write you a prescription if you want that.

Hormonal Diseases

If your period problems turn out to be an illness this section is for you. But there is only so much a book can offer. I'd recommend seeing a herbalist if you have one of these diagnosed by your doctor.

ENDOMETRIOSIS

Why do I have Endometriosis?

Getting diagnosed with Endometriosis or Adenomyosis is a lengthy process for most. Often it comes with a sigh of relief as you finally understand what is causing your pain. But sadly the treatment options for these diseases are sometimes as harsh as the illness itself. Having said that, there is a lot which can be done naturally to ease your symptoms too.

What is it?

Endometriosis (endo) and adenomyosis (adeno) are conditions where tissue which looks and behaves very similar to endometrial tissue is found somewhere other than inside the uterus. But the disease tissue is biochemically different to normal endometrial tissue (endometriosis-uk.org, 2018). Endometriotic implants have an over-expression of beta estrogen receptors. The two terms, endometriosis and adenomyosis, describe the location of said tissue. Adeno is when endomertrial-like tissue is found between the uterine muscles. Whereas, endometriosis is when endometrial-like tissue is found on the ovaries, fallopian tubes, outer wall of the uterus, the uterine or ovarian ligaments, bowel, ureters or bladder. Most of the symptoms associated with these conditions are because the endometrial-like tissue responds to the natural hormone cycle, bleeding each month. Sometimes the blood is surrounded by the body in a thick coating that traps the blood and becomes a "chocolate cyst". This will keep on growing and potentially burst at some point. But this is hard to predict. Careful monitoring is crucial and surgery recommended.

No one knows what causes it, and that makes it difficult to prevent. It's also not possible to predict the progression of these conditions, which makes it hard to decide on appropriate preventative treatments for yourself.

When does it happen?

Endometriosis affects between 10-15% of the population worldwide (Rogers et.al., 2009). It is the second most common gynaecological condition in the UK and could be the cause of up to 50% of cases of infertility (Meuleman, et.al., 2009). Interestingly, the amount of people diagnosed with endometriosis following a laparoscopy doubles when there is the intention of finding endometriosis. So it would seem, it is not easy to spot unless you are looking for it.

What does it feel like?

Both adeno and endo are painful conditions for most who know they have it. It can feel like a deep heavy dragging sensation in the abdomen but is often a sharp severe pain. Depending on where the endometrial tissue is it can also feel like IBS, cystitis and pelvic inflammatory disease. It is often accompanied by depression or anxiety.

Diagnosis

The only surefire way of knowing you have endometriosis or adenomyosis is by having a laproscopy. This is a process of key hole surgery where a camera is inserted into the abdominal cavity and tissue samples are taken. Interestingly, it's very hard to see any difference between actual endometrial tissue and endometriosis tissue.

Causes

No one really knows why endometriosis and adenomyosis occur. Some define it as an inflammatory illness, not a hormone condition. But, endometriosis and adenomyosis are related to relative oestrogen excess. This means oestrogen is either high or is unopposed by sufficient progesterone. This makes hormonal treatment difficult.

The relative oestrogen excess seems to fuel the growth of endometrial tissue outside of the uterus whereas it is progesterone that causes many of the symptoms, as it responds to progesterone in the luteal phase and bleeds. The rates of incidence of these conditions increases in women, who have more menstrual cycles than most each year, started their menses early and/or have not been pregnant.

One theory of causation is that blood from the period flows backwards thanks to a partial blockage at the cervix or hymen. But this backflow has been debunked as it is actually so common as to be called normal. A second theory is that the immune system, which usually stops the abnormal growth of endometrial tissue where it is not expected, is lowered which permits this to occur. Which means it may originate in the immune system.

Things you can do

Treatment options for adeno/endo usually involve trying to reduce oestrogen levels with contraceptive pills. Other treatment options are pain killers, antidepressants and finally surgery. In 62% of cases surgery will improve or resolve the problem. But sadly, 5 years after successful treatment most will have a recurrence. When I see a patient I listen to what their needs are to decide how to treat them. Usually the pain is top priority. Each patient will receive individualised blends depending on their symptoms and priorities. Some experience long cycles, some short, some very heavy, some very scanty. So it makes sense to have a selection of herbs which can deal with all of that.

Reducing oestrogen is like putting a bucket under a leaking roof. It doesn't fix the underlying problem, which could be stress, obesity, fatigue, poor eating habits, genetics or a combination of all of these. But there are a lot of things you can do for yourself which will complement your treatment.

If you're carrying a little extra weight you may be increasing your oestrogen levels without realising it. This is because fat cells make oestrogen. If your liver is struggling perhaps with the burdens of alcohol and caffeine it will need help to process the oestrogen in the body. Decreasing your stress will always improve your immunity and your immunity is quite likely compromised in endo/adeno, as the body is allowing tissue to grow where it should not. These things can be difficult to change, especially with diet. That's why I focus so much on helping people create diet plans that suit their lifestyle. Without that, it's hard to put things into action:

FOOD
» Be sure to eat a lot of fruit and vegetables. This is so that you're getting fibre that will help your bowels stay regular and limit the amount of oestrogen able to recirculate in the body.

HABIT
» Avoid plastic food packaging as this contains chemicals that promote oestrogen.

FOOD
» Eat organic meat, dairy, and eggs as animals reared non-organically can be fed lots of hormones during their lives which affect us when we eat them.

FOOD
» Avoid caffeine and alcohol because they tax the liver which is trying so hard to clear your body of oestrogen, why give it more to do?

FOOD
» Supplement with Vitamin E to reduce adhesions and scar tissue.

HABIT
» Exercise for 20 mins using a high intensity interval training workout from youtube. This improves your metabolism and circulation.

HABIT
» Avoid detergents and household cleaners with oestrogen derivatives.

FOOD
» Supplement with essential fatty acids (aka. fish or seed oils) as these reduce inflammatory prostaglandins which cause pain.

FOOD
» Avoid refined sugar and refined carbohydrates because they increase your insulin levels and put your hormones out of balance.

FOOD
» Eat citrus fruits and berries because they're high in Vitamin C and support the immune system in viewing the endometrial tissue as an unusual growth that should be broken down.

FOOD
» Eat foods which increase the breakdown of oestrogen: carrots, broccoli, beetroot, globe artichoke, brussels sprouts, cabbage, cauliflower, lemons, watercress, garlic, leeks and onions.

FOOD
» Eat fermented foods or supplement with a probiotic. It has been observed that women with endo or adeno have low lactobacillus levels in the gut flora.

The herbs

There are a lot of options when it comes to herbs. Not only are there various actions that we'd want to combine in a blend for the problem but also there are multiple herbs that have said action. I wouldn't recommend picking them at random without consulting a herbalist. I've included a safe option blend that will support the body without causing any potential problems. It's a gentle way to help you that won't have the same potency as getting a bespoke blend made. But at least it's somewhere to start if you have 0 monies.

» **Reduce pain:** white willow bark (*Salix alba*) or meadowsweet (*Filipendula ulmaria*)

» **Support the liver:** dandelion root (*Taraxacum officinalis rad.*) or milk thistle (*Carduus marianus*)

» **Cleanse, tone and heal the uterus:** lady's mantle (*Alchemilla vulgaris*) or raspberry leaf (*Rubus idaeus*)

» **Improve circulation:** hawthorn (*Crataegus spp.*) or cinnamon (*Cinnamomum zeylanicum*)

» **Increase immunity:** echinacea (*Echinacea spp.*) or marigold (*Calendula officinalis*)

» **Relax the body:** skullcap (*Scutellaria lateriflora*) or passionflower (*Passiflora incarnata*)

» **Reduce cortisol:** ashwagandha (*Withania somnifera*) or siberian ginseng (*Eleutherococcus senticosus*)

Endometriosis/Adenomyosis Herbal Tea
» Dandelion root (*Taraxacum officinale rad.*) 20g
» Raspberry leaf (*Rubus idaeus*) 10g
» Hawthorn (*Crataegus spp.*) 5g
» Marigold (*Calendula officinalis*) 5g
» Skullcap (*Scutellaria lateriflora*) 10g
» Ashwagandha (*Withania somnifera*) 20g
» White willow bark (*Salix alba*) 10g

Try this for a month by having a cup of tea 3 times a day, if things get worse stop immediately. If there is no improvement in 3 months, see a herbalist (or just see a herbalist from the start).

PCOS

Getting diagnosed with PCOS can be confusing. There are so many things which contribute to the problem – how do you know what to do? You might not like the options given to you for treatment either. We're still not sure why it happens, but looking at things like diet and lifestyle can shed more light than just thinking about it physically.

What is it?

Polycystic ovarian syndrome (PCOS) is a disorder of the endocrine system affecting 5–8% of the population (Azziz et.al. 2004). As the name implies it is characterised by many cysts being found inside the ovary. These are follicles which do not reach maturity but are greater than 20mm in size – known as ovarian cysts (Knight, 2017). It is normal for the ovary to contain many undeveloped follicles as the eggs stored there are in all stages of development at all times in a menstruating woman. It has been observed that 20% of women will have undeveloped follicles the right size to be considered cysts without any symptoms of illness (Trickey, 2003). Therefore, it could be considered normal or unpathological in some women.

It is more important to consider PCOS an illness of the endocrine system, perhaps even without the presence of polycystic ovaries but *always* accompanied by too much androgen and *usually* insulin resistance leading to irregular ovulation and menstruation. Only 7–8% of women with polycystic ovaries will have PCOS but 70–80% of women who don't ovulate will have PCOS (Trickey, 2003). 80% of women who have excessive hair growth and no changes to their period have PCOS. Therefore, PCOS has implications for fertility. It can increase your chances of cardiovascular disease too. But with some dietary and lifestyle changes it can be a perfectly manageable condition.

When does it happen?

PCOS can occur from the start of menstruation in the teen years and continue through life if left untreated.

What does it feel like?

It usually doesn't feel like anything aside from very frustrating! You might notice that you aren't having periods and you may be overweight, have acne and a male pattern of hair growth. Not everyone feels the same with it as there are a variety of presentations. Of those that have it:

» 90% have irregular cycles
» 80% don't ovulate
» 50–70% are insulin resistant
» 60% have excessive body hair
» 50% don't have periods
» 40% are overweight
» 30% have abnormal bleeds
» 15% don't see a change in their basal body temperature

Diagnosis

There are a few tests which are needed to confirm you have PCOS. Most doctors will start by testing the blood for elevated androgen levels. They will then do a fasting blood glucose level to see if you have insulin resistance. Finally, you should have an ultrasound scan done to confirm you have polycystic ovaries. A diagnosis is concluded upon when you're found to have a few of the following; polycystic ovaries, elevated androgen, irregular ovulation, male pattern hair, and/or elevated insulin levels.

Causes

Nobody really knows what causes PCOS but it usually arises from 1 of 2 things: diet or stress. Diet/genes and/or stress lead to insulin resistance and an over-production of androgens. It is usually considered an illness of insulin resistance, 50–70% of women with PCOS have this (Trickey, 2003). However, I have had patients who do not respond to an improvement in diet but rather to an improvement in their stress levels. This is because disturbances in cortisol (a key stress hormone) production has implications to our insulin regulation and therefore androgen production. Knowing whether diet or stress will be key for your treatment seems to be something which is only realised upon experimentation in both.

Some people are born with Type 1 diabetes and that can only ever be managed, not cured. But most will come to get Type 2 diabetes through a combination of genes, diet and life events. We know now that long term stress is linked to isulin resistance. Stress increases noradrenaline and cortisol. Noradrenaline reduces the body's ability to use insulin and cortisol increases insulin levels, therefore leading to insulin resistance. Being overweight also contributes to getting PCOS. The fat cells make androgen that increases testosterone and estron. This is fine in normal quantities but when they get excessive the estron competes with estradiol (which goes on to make oestrogen) and the testosterone competes with SHBG that controls how you use testosterone. So without SHBG giving testosterone instructions it floats around freely leading to the excessive hair and lack of periods.

Risk factors include; sedentary lifestyle, obesity, smoking, some diuretic drugs, corticosteroids, and perhaps some contraceptive pills.

Normal treatment

When you see a doctor they are likely to offer a few drugs because they want to treat it from many angles. They are likely to use a drug to treat the insulin resistance (usually metformin), a drug to ensure a regular period (usually the contraceptive pill), a drug to treat the effects of excessive androgen (such as androcur) and something to improve fertility when that becomes an issue (often clomid). The natural options seek to do the same thing, just go about it a little differently.

Things you can do

One of the hardest things about getting diagnosed with PCOS is how it affects the rest of your health, not just your reproductive organs. The options you're given for treatment might not be what you want to take or you might have tried them and found they didn't work.

When I see a patient I listen to what their needs are to decide how to treat them. Usually excessive hair and acne are top priority, or infertility if they're trying for a baby. You can see that there is a lot of variation with PCOS. No two women will suffer in the same way. So it makes sense to have a selection of herbs that can deal with all of that. Just reducing androgens is like putting a bucket under a leaking roof. It doesn't fix the underlying problem, which could be stress, obesity, fatigue, poor eating habits, genetics or a combination of all of these. There is however, a lot that can be done with diet and lifestyle alone. Arguably, the dietary changes should make the back bone of any PCOS treatment as many women manage their PCOS with just diet and lifestyle changes.

Eating low glycemic load foods such as whole grains, fresh fruit and vegetables is crucial to lose weight. These foods are sustaining and don't create big peaks and troughs in your blood sugar (unless you binge on fruit juice). The 5:2 diet where you have 2 days a week that are "fasting" days will also help you reset your insulin resistance. There are tons of books available now which focus on recipes for fasting days. You can ease yourself into it too if you're scared about getting hypoglycaemic episodes. The fasting days are not days where you eat nothing, but rather you are allowed 800 calories as a woman. That can be quite a lot of food if it's all natural whole foods. Here's a list of low glycemic load foods to concentrate on eating, as well as good habits to start practising:

FOOD
» Supplement with essential fatty acids (aka. fish or seed oils).

FOOD
» Avoid refined sugar and refined carbohydrates because these increase your insulin levels and put your hormones out of balance.

FOOD
» Be sure to eat fibre-rich foods like vegetables, fruit and legumes as these increase shbg.

HABIT
» Exercise for 20 mins using a high interval training workout from youtube. This improves your metabolism and circulation.

HABIT
» Avoid detergents and household cleaners with oestrogen derivatives.

FOOD
» Supplement with Vitamin C, 500mg twice a day to boost immunity which is compromised in insulin resistance.

FOOD
» Supplement with magnesium 400–800mg and chromium 200–800mg to help regulate your blood sugar levels.

FOOD
» Supplement with B-complex to manage stress levels and improve immunity.

FOOD
» Eat foods which aid the liver to break down excessive hormones: carrots, broccoli, sprouts, globe artichoke, fennel, lemon and watercress.

FOOD

» Take a probiotic each day if you're having problems with recurring thrush.

FOOD

» Supplement with zinc, 20mg to support the endocrine system and balance blood sugar.

The herbs

There are a lot of options when it comes to herbs. Not only are there various actions that we'd want to combine in a blend for the problem but there are multiple herbs which have said action. I wouldn't recommend picking them at random without consulting a herbalist. I've included a safe option blend that will support the body without causing any potential problems. It's a gentle way to help you that won't have the same potency as getting a bespoke blend made. But at least it's somewhere to start if you have o monies. Losing weight is one of the hardest challenges we face and that's because our lifestyles don't support natural, healthy eating habits. We have unpredictable diaries or long days where it's all too easy to reach for the sugar hit to keep working.

» **Balance blood sugar levels:** dandelion root (*Taraxacum officinalis rad.*) or cinnamon (*Cinnamomum zeylanicum*)

» **Reduce androgens:** spearmint (*Mentha spicata*) or peony (*Paeonia lactiflora*)

» **Improve liver function:** dandelion root (*Taraxacum officinalis rad.*)

» **Protect circulation:** hawthorn (*Crataegus spp.*)

» **Increase immunity:** echinacea (*Echinacea spp.*)

» **Reduce anxiety:** skullcap (*Scutellaria lateriflora*) or passionflower (*Passiflora incarnata*)

» **Reduce cortisol:** ashwagandha (*Withania somnifera*) or siberian ginseng (*Eleutherococcus senticosus*)

PCOS herbal tea

- » Dandelion root (*Taraxacum officinale rad.*) 20g
- » Spearmint (*Mentha spicata*) 10g
- » Hawthorn (*Crataegus spp.*) 10g
- » Globe artichoke (*Cynara scolymus*) 10g
- » Skullcap (*Scutellaria lateriflora*) 10g
- » Ashwagandha (*Withania somnifera*) 20g

Try this for a month by having a cup of tea 3 times a day. If things get worse stop immediately. If there is no improvement in 3 months, see a herbalist – or, again, just see a herbalist from the start.

FIBROIDS

Getting diagnosed with a foreign mass growing inside you isn't the most comforting of things to hear. But it's not as bad as it sounds, because there are treatment options that don't involve surgery. Nobody really knows why they happen but looking at things like diet and lifestyle can shed more light than just thinking about it physically.

What is it?

Fibroids are non-cancerous tumours of the uterus. They vary in size, position and quantity for each individual woman. They can be as small as a pea and sometimes large enough that you look 6 or 7 months pregnant. They are made of dense muscular fibre which is arranged in circular layers and covered in a layer of compressed smooth muscle. A fibroid doesn't have much blood flow inside it but rather it is supplied blood from the outside. When fibroids grow quickly they are linked to sarcoma but when this is observed they are removed before it becomes a more serious issue.

Where does it happen?

There are 3 types of fibroid: intrauterine, myometrial, and extrauterine, depending on where they are in relation to the uterus. An intrauterine or submucosal fibroid is within the uterine cavity and is usually smaller than 5–6 cms. They can usually be removed through a hysteroscope. They interfere with endometrial growth wherever it is in the uterus. This can make implantation of a fertilised egg difficult and lower fertility. A myometrial or submucosal fibroid is within the uterus muscles. It can put pressure on the bowel, bladder or kidney. These fibroids can lower fertility if they grow into the uterus. The final type of position is an extrauterine or subserous one. These grow on the outside of the uterus but they can also grow on the fallopian tubes.

When does it happen?

Fibroids are more common later in life, 20–25% of women over 35 will have one / some at some point (Trickey, 2003).

What does it feel like?

Sometimes fibroids don't feel like anything at all and are found by tests being done for other reasons. But usually they create heavy periods and a dragging sensation in the pelvis. Sometimes they interfere with fertility and that can be how they come to be diagnosed. If they grow large enough or are in a particular position they will start to push on other organs and create problems there too. They can cause constipation by pressing on the bowel, or you may find you need to pee all the time as they decrease the capacity of the bladder. Occasionally they press in such a way that the kidneys get into trouble, but this is rare.

Diagnosis

The best way to find out if you have fibroids is to have an ultrasound. This is totally non invasive and very precise. It will usually be able to tell you how many there are, where they are and how large they are. Of course, you might just have the one. Sometimes doctors will advise that you get a laparoscopy if a fibroid is tricky to see on an ultrasound.

Causes

Nobody really knows why exactly fibroids grow in the first place. We do know that they almost always start to decrease in size or stop growing when oestrogen is taken out of the picture. This doesn't mean that there is necessarily too much oestrogen in the system, it usually means that there is *relatively* too much in the system. By this I mean that other hormones that normally help to counterbalance oestrogen are so low the symptoms of too much oestrogen take hold. There are some things that increase your risk of getting them though: coffee, hypertension, using perineal talcum powder and obesity. Pregnancies reduce your risk and (ironically enough) smoking seems to as well. Though, of course, that's in no way a recommendation to start smoking. It isn't yet clear if hormonal contraceptives help or hinder when it comes to the likelihood of getting fibroids.

Normal treatment

Fibroids don't always need treatment if they are small enough and don't cause many symptoms. They can be left alone with regular monitoring to see if they are growing. If they do cause symptoms you will probably have been offered surgery and perhaps medications that will reduce your oestrogen levels as well. But there are a lot more options available to you when it comes to natural remedies and herbs.

Things you can do

One of the hardest things about getting diagnosed with fibroids is feeling like you have no options. Often you're told to go home and not worry about it. But that's not very comforting. When I get ill I want to know everything I can do to help the situation improve. When I see a patient I listen to what their needs are to decide how to treat them. Usually heavy periods are top priority, along with the dragging, uncomfortable sensation that the presence of the fibroid is causing.

You can see that fibroids come in a variety of sizes and locations that can create a variety of symptoms. So it makes sense to have a selection of herbs that can deal with all of that. Reducing oestrogen is like putting a bucket under a leaking roof. It doesn't fix the underlying problem, which could be stress, obesity, fatigue, poor eating habits, genetics or a combination of all of these:

FOOD

» Be sure to eat a lot of fresh fruit and vegetables. This is so that you're getting fibre, which will help your bowels stay regular. If you have a fibroid which is interfering with your ability to go regularly you may find your body starts to suffer with a backlog of toxins. Try taking swedish bitters, prune juice or dandelion coffee to start your day.

HABIT

» Avoid plastic food packaging as this contains chemicals which promote oestrogen.

FOOD

» Eat organic meat, dairy, and eggs as animals reared non-organically can be fed lots of hormones during their lives which affect us when we eat them.

FOOD

» Avoid caffeine and alcohol because they tax the liver which is trying so hard to clear your body of oestrogen, why give it more to do?

FOOD

» Supplement with Vitamin E – we're not sure why this works but it does.

HABIT

» Exercise for 20 mins using a high intensity interval training workout from youtube. This improves your metabolism and circulation.

HABIT

» Avoid detergents and household cleaners with oestrogen derivatives.

FOOD

» Supplement with essential fatty acids (aka. fish or seed oils). Avoid refined sugar and refined carbohydrates because they increase your insulin levels and put your hormones out of balance.

FOOD

» Eat citrus fruits and berries because they're high in Vitamin C and support the immune system in viewing the fibroid as an unusual

growth which should be broken down.

FOOD

» Take an iron supplement. If you have heavy periods it's important to supplement with iron in a natural way. Try taking floradix, this will improve iron levels, won't add to constipation and will help you lose less blood next month round.

FOOD

» Eat foods which increase the breakdown of oestrogen: carrots, broccoli, beetroot, globe artichoke, brussels sprouts, cabbage, cauliflower, lemons, watercress, garlic, leeks and onions.

The herbs

There are a lot of options when it comes to herbs. I've included a safe option blend that will support the body without causing any potential problems. It's a gentle way to help you that won't have the same potency as getting a bespoke blend made. But at least it's somewhere to start if you have o monies.

» **Support the liver:** dandelion root (*Taraxacum officinalis rad.*) or milk thistle (*Carduus marianus*)

» **Cleanse, tone and heal the uterus:** lady's mantle (*Alchemilla vulgaris*) or raspberry leaf (*Rubus idaeus*)

» **Increase circulation:** hawthorn (*Crataegus spp*) or cinnamon (*Cinnamomum zeylanicum*)

» **Increase immunity:** echinacea (*Echinacea spp.*)
» **Relax the body:** chamomile (*Chamomilla recutita*) or vervain (*Verbena officinalis*)
» **Reduce cortisol:** ashwagandha (*Withania somnifera*) or siberian ginseng (*Eleutherococcus senticosus*)

Fibroid Herbal Tea
» Dandelion root (*Taraxacum officinale rad.*) 20g
» Lady's mantle (*Alchemilla vulgaris*) 10g
» Hawthorn (*Crataegus spp.*) 10g
» Echinacea root (*Echinacea spp.*) 10g
» Chamomile (*Chamomilla recutita*) 10g
» Ashwagandha (*Withania somnifera*) 20g

Try this for a month by having a cup of tea 3 times a day. If things get worse stop immediately. If there is no improvement in 3 months, see a herbalist, or just see a herbalist from the start.

Part Two

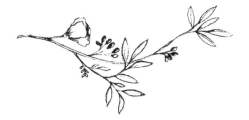

Wellness   Problem   Illness

The Herbs

HOW TO CHOOSE HERBS THAT ARE RIGHT FOR YOU

Before we talk recipes, let's first cover how to choose the *right* herb or recipe for you.

It's all too common for me to see people turning to google for advice on period problems. It's not easy to get an appointment with the right person in the NHS anymore (in the UK) and so more and more people try to find answers for themselves. But just like you've heard before, Doctor Google is not your friend. I would always recommend a written reference such as *Bartram's Encyclopedia of Herbal Medicine* to aid you instead.

But remember that a diagnosis is the first hurdle for any problem. Even if you're totally against the drugs offered to you by the doctor, it's well worth going just to find out what is *really* going on. As harmless as herbs generally are, if used incorrectly they can add to a problem, rather than improve things.

Step 1

Whenever you have a health complaint the first thing to do is to keep a record. Start by creating a table with the days of the month along the top and a list of symptoms down the left side. Rate each symptom on a 1–5 scale each day for a month. This will give you a clear idea if the issue is cycling with your menstruation or more common than that. It's at this stage you could see a doctor to start the support process.

Step 2

Once you've got a record of the symptoms over one menstrual cycle turn to your books. Look up the symptom and see what herbs come up. I'd recommend *Bartram's Encyclopaedia* (as mentioned above) or Anne McIntyre's *Women's Book of Herbs* and of course, the back of this book. You'll usually get a selection of around 5 herbs to choose from.

Step 3

Now look up each of these herbs individually and read through all the uses they have. You might find that some treat problems you've had in the past too. Generally speaking, the more things a herb treats which you have currently or have had in the past, the more likely it is to suit your constitution. Rate them from most fitting to last and source the best-fitted herb on that list. If you are in the UK I'd recommend using online shops such as Neal's Yard Remedies, or Baldwin's, for this.

Step 4

Take this herb for your next cycle. If you're using a tea take 3 cups of tea each day using a teaspoon of herb each time. If using a tincture, take 3ml 3 times a day.

Step 5

Go back to your record and begin again for this month. By the end of it you will be able to compare two menstrual cycles. This is the best possible way to know how a herb is affecting you. Generally the longer the problem has been going on, the longer you will need to continue with the herb. I usually treat a patient for a minimum of 3 months. 1 month to see if I have the right herbs, 2 months to see if it was all just a fluke, and 3 months to confirm it was definitely the herbs helping and to establish a pattern. After the third month I usually try giving the patient a break for 2–4 weeks to see if the symptoms return. If I have the right herbs and the problem is fairly simple and the patient hasn't had it for centuries it usually does the trick. If it doesn't then we try another 3 months on it before considering a rest. It's important to keep trying to come off the herbs, otherwise you may be taking them for no reason without knowing you're actually feeling better.

Herbs shouldn't be used like a bucket under a leaking roof unless it's urgent. They can help the body patch the leak forever and do not need to be used ad infinitum.

Kitchen sink technique

I prefer everyone to just try a single herb at a time. That way if it doesn't work you know exactly what it was and can move on to the next herb on your list. But I admit this is a pretty long-winded methodology, it could take you 3 months just to find out that 3 different herbs don't help. So sometimes it's better to go with the "kitchen sink" approach and bung it all in. I don't have a problem with this so long as you're not wasting your money and don't have a bad reaction to the blend. If you have a bad reaction it's hard to know which of the herbs was causing the issue.

The recipes I have given on the following pages should be thought of as a single entity. Once herbs are combined, they blend in synergistic harmony to become another thing entirely. So while you can choose a blend of herbs, I would still only try one blend at a time so you can still isolate it if you need to take it out of your regime later on.

It is very tempting to try a nutritional supplement with a new therapy and a couple of herbal recipes. But try not to, you might end up feeling you need to take 5 different things when actually only 1 of them is the one that is working. If it's so serious that you feel inclined to use ALL the remedies, I implore you to see a herbalist.

Where to find a herbalist

You can see a herbalist from my team at Forage Botanicals if the problem suits online consultations. Alternatively, in the UK you can find trained herbalists through the National Institute of Medical Herbalists or the Unified Register of Herbalists' website.

Where to get your herbs

I'd recommend getting herbs in the UK from Baldwin's, Neal's Yard Remedies or Starchild online. They both get their herbs mostly from organic, British suppliers, as far as I'm aware from having worked at Neal's Yard for 7 years.

If you're in America then I hear Rose Mountain Herbs are a great online stockist.

I don't recommend buying herbs already in capsules if you can help it because you miss out on the healing communicated through taste, and it's easier for contamination to occur. A few years back there was an issue with St. John's Wort pills from a nationwide pharmacy in the UK. St. John's Wort got all the terrible press when in fact there had actually been a contaminate in it that had caused the health complications in those taking them.

If you buy dried herbs or tinctures from the people I recommend you'll get a better relationship with the plants and the chances of them being contaminated, or the wrong plant altogether, are very small.

Warning: You MUST check all of these herbs for their safety at the back of the book, and don't experiment without seeing a specialist if you are already taking medication. I have specifically chosen herbs that have little to no safety issues, but you still need to do your research first before taking them.

Recipes

INFUSIONS AND DECOCTIONS

An infusion is pretty much what you'd expect to do to a tea. You simply pour boiling water over dried herbs and let it infuse, then strain it before drinking. A decoction, on the other hand, will be less familiar. A decoction is made by putting dried herb material into cold water in a pan on the stove, bringing to boiling point and simmering for 10 minutes. Then it is strained and served. Generally speaking decoctions are best used with roots and barks, whereas infusions are used for leaves and flowers.

Night time tea

- » Passionflower
- » Rose
- » Lemonbalm

This remedy is for anyone who believes that stress is contributing to their problem, especially if you are in stage 1 of stress and feeling pretty anxious. It will also help with long-term stress (stage 2 or 3) but it's likely to need to be taken alongside adaptogens such as the recipe below this for that. If you're going through short-term stress try this first.

Recipe

- » **40g passionflower** (*Passiflora incarnata*). A slightly trippy, dreamlike plant, it is a relaxant and helps with short-term stress, anxiety and insomnia.

» **10g rose** (*Rosa damascena*), a herb of love. It helps you to love yourself enough to take time out. To lessen the metaphorical load you bear on your back or maybe even ask for help!

» **50g lemonbalm** (*Melissa officinalis*), a relaxant that has an uplifting cheerful quality. It also calms the heart and tummy so if you're feeling nerves in your tummy or experiencing palpitations this is the herb for you.

How to use

Combine these herbs. If this tea works for you, you should feel instantly calmer upon tasting it. Have a cup an hour before bed. This should allow you to pee before bed without being woken in the night for the same reason. Take this tea every day whilst feeling stressed.

Adrenal fatigue recovery decoction

» Nettle seed
» Liquorice
» Rhemmania

Adrenal fatigue is what happens in stage 3 stress. It is usually a result of long-term stress which has become so normalised the fatigue really takes you by surprise. It's likely that you may have stopped having periods or are suffering with irregular cycles if you are adrenally fatigued, as you've been making enough cortisol to steal from your progesterone reserves.

All the herbs in this recipe are what are called adaptogenic. They help your body adapt to stress, reduce the recovery time and improve your stamina and immunity while at it.

Recipe

- » **20g nettle** (*Urtica dioica*) seed. This is one of very few native adaptogens to the UK. It is a firey herb that can sometimes overstimulate. If you find this blend makes you more wired than before, I'd try just oat tops (*Avena sativa*) instead. It is a nerve tonic rather than an adaptogen and probably what you need for a while before moving on to nettle seed.

- » **10g liquorice** (*Glycyrrhiza glabra*). Liquorice is 1000 times sweeter than sugar and adds a sweetness to this mix. It is an adaptogen which supports the lungs and digestion as well. Aiding with asthma and constipation.

- » **80g rhemmania** (*Rhemmania glutinosa*). This is is an adaptogen from China. When I was fatigued I used a special chinese preparation called fermented rhemmania (*Shu Di Huang*). It looks completely black and is very chewy. I found the taste incredibly nourishing at the time. Now that I don't need it I don't find the smell or taste enticing at all. Whichever preparation you are able to find, it will build up energy resources when you're totally depleted.

How to use

Put 2 teaspoons of this blend in a litre of cold water. Place in a pan and bring to the boil on the stove. Simmer this for 15 mins with a lid on before straining. Drink this litre of decoction through the day either hot or cold. Repeat this each day for a month. For a super-strong decoction, leave the herbs to soak overnight before bringing to boil in the morning.

Anxiety relief tea

- » Liquorice
- » Lime blossom
- » Hawthorn blossom or berry

If you're a worrier it's important to nourish yourself. Take time to slow down and lessen the amount you feel you're dealing with. Get help with your workload too, so it doesn't feel like it's all on you.

I find when I'm anxious that keeping moving is important. If I sit or lie down in one place for a long time my mind will just go around in circles. A walk in nature or a swim does it for me. These herbs support the nerves and nourish the adrenals for anxiety relief during the day minus any drowsiness.

Recipe

- » **20g liquorice** (*Glycyrrhiza glabra*). Liquorice supports the adrenal glands, and when you downregulate the adrenals, you tend to feel less like your mind is spiralling into a pit of despair. (Can you tell anxiety is something I've dealt with?!)

- » **40g lime blossom** (*Tilia cordata*). This is a beautifully delicate blossom, which grows on the big, strong lime trees across the UK. It is a relaxant, especially useful for those who give out more energy than they take back for themselves, the serial helpers.

- » **40g hawthorn** (*Crataegus spp.*). Hawthorn isn't well known for its actions against anxiety, but I find it indispensable for this use. It's more famously known for its strengthening abilities on the heart. But anyone who's experienced anxiety before can see how something that supports the heart would be desirable!

How to use

Use a teaspoon of the blend in a cup of boiled water. Let it infuse for 10 mins before drinking. Have a cup of this infusion (tea) as often as you require it but at least once a day till the anxiety is gone.

Heavy period protection decoction

» Nettle
» Raspberry
» Lady's mantle

The herbs in this blend help nourish the blood but also stop any excess bleeding. I once had a patient who had been bleeding non-stop for 15 days when she came to see me. She was perimenopausal and I gave her a blend that included these herbs. Within a day the bleeding stopped. I would expect heavy blood flow to stop within 5 days of taking these herbs if started whilst on a period. But the effects of the blood building herb (nettle) will only be felt over a longer time period, say a month.

Recipe

» **50g nettle** (*Urtica dioica*). This is the blood builder I speak of. It is rich in iron along with vitamins A, B, C, D, and K, making it a flipping great superfood! By building up your iron stores you reduce the amount you're likely to lose for the next period.

» **50g raspberry** (*Rubus idaeus*) or lady's mantle (*Alchemilla vulgaris*) Both are drying herbs (haemostatic). They will stop excessive blood flow in a pinch.

How to use

Combine these in equal parts. You can prepare these as an infusion or as a decoction. A decoction is stronger.

For a decoction put a tablespoon of the combined herbs to soak in a litre of cold water over night. Bring to the boil in a pan in the morning. Simmer for 10 mins and strain. Drink throughout the day.

For an infusion use a teaspoon for each cup of tea you make. Pour on boiled water; infuse for 10 mins, then strain. Repeat this three times a day.

Drink the decoction or infusion each day for a month.

Nervous tummy tea

- » Marshmallow root
- » Chamomile
- » Peppermint

Recipe

- » **40g marshmallow** (*Althea officinalis*) root, a gentle demulcent. It coats the digestion in lovely gloopy stuff that helps it feel warm, comforted and protected.

- » **40g chamomile** (*Chamomilla recutita*), a relaxant on the nerves and digestion. It also relieves spasm.

- » **20g peppermint** (*Mentha piperita*). Peppermint is another anti-spasmodic but it has a contradictory stimulating nature that makes it good for staying alert in the day too. There is a mahoosive nerve – the vagus nerve – which connects your brain with your gut. So it's not a surprise that when we're feeling anxious we can often find ourselves rushing for the bathroom. The herbs in this recipe both calm and soothe the digestion.

How to use

Use a teaspoon of the blend in a cup of boiled water. Let it infuse for 10 mins before drinking. Have a cup of this infusion (tea) as often as you require.

BATH POTIONS

Who doesn't love a good bath? Only very strange people I say!

Geranium shea butter melt

This recipe is a hormone balancing treat to help stress, PMS, depression and anxiety levels. It may become part of your new self-care routine. Having something homemade and special to use makes us feel loved, an important part of any healing.

Recipe

- » **3 drops geranium** (*Pelargonium graveolens*). This is a fabulous sweet-smelling essential oil. It doesn't take much to totally overpower whatever you're blending it with so BEWARE. In this instance it's just plain so won't cause problems, but do go easy on the dose. It is wonderful for balancing the hormones. I find it rather cheerful too.

- » **25g shea butter** – this is a beautiful natural butter which moisturises the skin and smells good enough to eat.

How to use

Melt 25g shea butter in a bain marie or double boiler and add 3 drops of Geranium essential oil, mix, then pour into silicone moulds (which are suitable for chocolate making). Leave these to solidify before popping them out. It's often best to store these in the fridge so they stay solid. Simply add one to each bath as required. It'll melt, releasing the beautiful oil scent and the shea butter will moisturise your skin (and your bath). Beware of a slippery exit from said bath. Enjoy whenever you need it.

Clary sage and lavender bath salts

These salts are designed to help soothe the senses and relax your muscles during period pain or in the premenstrual phase when feeling a bit irritable.

Recipe

> » **3 drops clary sage** (*Salvia sclarea*). This essential oil is another herb that balances the hormones. It's most famous for helping with pain during labour and shouldn't be used during pregnancy because of that.

> » **5 drops lavender** (*Lavandula angustifolia*) essential oil – this is an oil I was basically raised on. My mum used it on everything. In this instance though it's for helping with relaxation.

> » **100g Epsom salts.** These are rich in magnesium, which is helpful for releasing cramps and muscle tension.

How to use

Use 100g of salts and add 5 drops lavender oil and 3 drops clary sage oil to it in a bowl. Mix well. Once combined you can add this to the bath as it runs and let it dissolve. I use 100g in each of my baths so just multiply this by however many baths worth you'd like to make at a time. You can store it in a glass jar by the bath to retain the smell. Just avoid keeping it in direct sunlight. This can be used whenever you wish, but is especially useful in the premenstrual and menstrual phase.

Chamomile, rose and oat bath sock

This soak is wonderful if you ever get dry or irritated skin. The oats create a milky consistency to the hot water and can leave the skin feeling silky smooth.

Recipe

- » **25g chamomile** (*Chamomilla recutita*) – used here not just to relax but also for its skin soothing abilities. It even helps abate itching.

- » **10g rose.** Rose (*Rosa damascena*), a gorgeous comforting herb that looks pretty. Who doesn't want prettiness in their bath?

- » **25g porridge oats.** These help to soothe the skin and will moisturise dry skin. If you put it all in a sock you can then rub it over the skin too. It's ideal for eczema.

How to use

Just mix together the ingredients in a bowl. Spoon the blend into a sock and tie it up. Add this to your bath water while it runs or tie it over the hot tap for the strongest infusion. Bathe with this sock of herbs in the bath. P.s. your sock will be ruined so it's best to use one of those old odd socks we all have lying around. Use this as required.

AROMATHERAPY

Antidepressant pulse point

- » Rose
- » Neroli
- » Sandalwood

It can be hard for some menstruators to avoid depression each month. As the hormones change in the premenstrual phase we naturally look inwards and can feel cut off. For others looking inwards is a bit too painful. I've even known women who are naturally very insular and end up feeling depressed during their ovulatiory phase because this phase asks them to go out and be social, which they don't really enjoy. Using comforting essential oils can help take the edge off when our hormones get us down.

Recipe

» **2 drops rose** (*Rosa damascena*) This is a comforting and antidepressing essential oil.

» **2 drops neroli** (*Citrus aurantium*) essential oil. This is another antidepressing oil. It's mentioned in this book as a dried herb under the name orange blossom.

» **5 drops sandalwood** (*Santalum album*). As an essential oil this is a calming grounding oil.

» **20ml base oil** (almond, sunflower, whatever you prefer). This is a scentless cheap oil which allows the essential oils to be applied to the skin safely without a skin reaction (unless you happen to be allergic of course).

How to use

Add 2 drops of rose, 2 drops of neroli and 5 drops of sandalwood essential oil to 20ml of base oil. It's easiest to use this if you can then pour it into an empty pulsepoint roller ball applicator. If you can't source those then put it into a glass dropper bottle that has a pipette in its lid. Simply apply a drop to the wrist, or roll on as required.

Anti-anxiety hanky insta-comfort

» Frankincense
» Marjoram

The hanky-method is how my mum used to give us essential oils for the day when we had exams. She'd simply put a few drops on a tissue and tuck it in our pocket. It's perfect if you can't apply oils to the skin or need something more subtle than rubbing stuff on.

Recipe

> » **5 drops frankincense** (*Boswellia serata*). As an essential oil, this helps us open the bronchioles and breathe deeper. This in turn makes us feel relaxed and is possibly why Catholic churches make me feel so zen.

> » **5 drops marjoram** (*Origanum majorana*). This essential oil is a relaxant that calms the nervous system; a lovely herbaceous smell that complements frankincense well.

How to use

Just put 5 drops of frankincense and marjoram onto a hanky or tissue for the day. Smell it whenever you need a calming moment.

Cramp massage oil

I have found stroking my stomach very soothing and distracting when I'm experiencing period pain. As oils are so easily absorbed through the skin I figured – why not add a massage oil into castor oil. It's a traditional remedy for period pain but if you can't find it use sunflower instead. Castor oil is quite sticky so you might prefer sunflower anyhow.

Recipe

> » **70ml sunflower oil** as a cheap readily available carrier oil.

» **10 drops peppermint** (*Mentha piperita*) essential oil for it's antispasmodic effects, easing muscular cramps.

» **10 drops lavender** (*Lavandula angustifolia*) essential oil as it is a gentle relaxant.

How to use
Mix the ingredients together and apply a pea sized amount to the hands then rub into the abdomen, thighs or back depending where you feel your period pain. Add more as required.

TINCTURES

Womb attunement

» Lady's mantle
» Rose

The womb often goes unattended to. It's as if it's a silent organ, hidden in the crevices, unfamiliar and unheard. Considering how much it really affects our daily lives, we aren't taught much about it. How have we so successfully removed the womb from our consciousness? Men are far more familiar with their testicles than we are our ovaries. Society teaches us to shrug off our hormonal changes, sexualises the vagina as a one-purpose-only penis-sheath. A lot of women have never looked at their vaginas.

Even I believe this disconnect of our bodies from our wombs leaves us weaker and more likely to get illnesses which affect this area as the womb cries out for attention.

By tuning into our wombs we reconnect with ourselves again. I have found this to have a plethora of benefits: from a renewed sense of sexuality to less pain during periods. I make a blend called Goddess drops, which is usually made up of lady's mantle, rose, mugwort and raspberry leaf, however here I've simplified it for you.

Recipe

- » **15ml rose** (*Rosa damascenca*). Rose tincture is associated with the Goddess Aphrodite. It is a herb of love and romance. It teaches us to love ourselves again.

- » **15ml lady's mantle** (*Alchemilla vulgaris*). This tincture is associated with the Goddess Virgin Mary. It is a herb which protects women as the Virgin Mary protected her disciples. It helps to bring the loving energy of rose to the womb.

How to use

Combine and take 3 drops on the tongue morning and night till the mix is finished. You'll be feeling like a Goddess in no time.

Insomnia b gone

- » Oat tops
- » Elderflower
- » Maybe valerian too

Insomnia can be quite scary. We all know how important sleep is, so to go without is unnerving. There are two reasons I find people can't sleep. Either they are full of cortisol / anxiety from the day, or they are so exhausted they don't have enough energy to engage in the act of sleep. This blend is best suited for people who are feeling wired or anxious from their day. I'd recommend using the adaptogenic mix in the tea section if you're in the "too tired to sleep situation" (it'll take a while for that to kick in if you need that).

Recipe

- » **20ml oat** (*Avena sativa*) tops. This tincture is a wonderfully soothing nervine. It coats the nervous system as though you are being wrapped in bubble wrap. Just what you need when you're strung out.

» **10ml elderflower** (*Sambucus nigra flos.*). This tincture isn't best known for helping with sleep but there are folk tales around falling asleep beneath an elder tree and being pulled into the land of the fae (a bit like Alice in Wonderland). I used this blend once on a strung out, overtired student and she said she slept like a baby.

» If these two herbs don't work then add 10ml of valerian, a strong sedative.

How to use
Combine and take 10ml before bed each night and 5ml in the mornings till your insomnia subsides.

Premenstrual lethargy pick-me-up

» Nettle seed
» Rosemary
» Nettle

One of the biggest period "pains" people complain of to me is lethargy, specifically in their premenstrual phase. This is the phase where energy naturally drops, so when you're working to your maximum every day the natural drop can hit you like a tonne of bricks. If you're unable to rest (which you should prioritise) this tincture will help give you a lift for the day. But make sure you prioritise some serious downtime as soon as possible. In fact, I'd recommend considering if there is anything in your daily life which can be reduced or delegated.

Recipe

» **80ml nettle** (*Urtica dioica*) seed tincture (can be left out if you can't find it), an excellent adaptogen full of firey Mars energy.

- » **15ml rosemary** (*Rosmarianus officinalis*) tincture, a stimulant to the circulation and brain.

- » **80ml nettle** (*Urtica dioica*) leaf tincture, a nourishing tonic, also full of firey Mars energy.

How to use

Combine and take 15ml as required. Don't exceed 45ml in a day. If it's not working by then, it's urgent that you get some rest!

Uplift my mood

- » Lemonbalm
- » Peppermint
- » Elderflower
- » Rose

For a gentle pick me up to the energy and mood this blend is lush. Lemonbalm and rose are known as herbal hugs in my herbie world. Peppermint and elderflower lift the spirit and energy, helping us feel a spring in our step.

Recipe

- » **20ml lemonbalm** (*Melissa officinalis*). This tincture is my favourite antidepressing herb. It lifts the mood and supports the digestion too.

- » **20ml rose** (*Rosa damascena*). This helps to bring a loving glow to any blend.

- » **20ml peppermint** (*Mentha piperita*). This tincture has a lovely upwards movement thanks to it's essential oils and helps add some zing to the blend.

- » **20ml elderflower** (*Sambucus nigra flos.*). Elderflower is a gentle mood improver full of the summer sun, when it's harvested.

How to use

Combine equal parts of each tincture and take 5ml three times each day for a month if this is a long-term low mood, or take 10ml as required for the occasional day.

Eliminate

- » Dandelion root
- » Chamomile
- » Burdock root
- » Cleavers

You have probably noticed that I mentioned the importance of supporting the liver in most of the period problems in this book. This advice is given on the basis that many hormone problems are worsened by a sluggish liver that is struggling to eliminate the hormones once they're done with them. This means that the hormones can circulate for longer and elongate their life in the body. This blend is for anyone thinking they could do with improving their liver function. It will be especially useful to anyone struggling with hormonal skin issues.

Recipe

- » **20ml dandelion root** (*Taraxacum officinalis rad.*). This tincture is to improve the speed of elimination and absorption of nutrients through an increase of bile production.

- » **30ml chamomile** (*Chamomilla recutita*) tincture, because it is a subtle bitter which helps soften the body and allow better absorption.

- » **20ml burdock** (*Arctium lappa rad.*) root tincture, as it is wonderful for assimilation, healing the gut wall and improving liver function.

» **30ml cleavers** (*Galium aperine*) tincture because it supports the lymphatic system which is another massive elimination pathway in the body.

How to use

Combine the ingredients and take 10ml each day for a month. Continue if it seems to be working and stop after 3 months to see if the problem returns. This blend can't be used in the luteal phase if you're trying to conceive.

Circulation stimulant

» Rosemary
» Ginger
» Cinnamon

In traditional herbal medicine we view good circulation as crucial to a healthy period. This blend is particularly relevant if you tend to be a cold person, have cold extremities, if all your heat tends to move away from your stomach when you bleed or if you have clots or light periods.

Recipe

» **20ml rosemary** (*Rosmarianus officinalis*). This tincture stimulates circulation by opening the blood vessels. It also supports memory and brain function.

» **5ml ginger** (*Zingiber officinale*) tincture, as it's so hot and helps boost circulation. It also supports digestion.

» **20ml cinnamon** (*Cinnamomum zeylanicum*) tincture. This is a warming herb that also boosts the metabolism.

How to use

Combine and take 10 drops in a little water morning and evening for a month. If it seems to be working then continue for 3 months before experimenting with stopping it.

It's all on me

- » Lime blossom
- » Rose
- » Liquorice
- » Hawthorn

If you've got a to-do list that barely fits on a piece of paper you're probably feeling like it's all on your shoulders. It's really important to delegate and prioritise if this is the case. I like to organise my to-do list by priority and then start putting the tasks into my calendar with an assigned amount of time for each task. There are only so many hours in the day after all, so there's no point having a list that seems infinitesimally large, as it really will never get done.

Recipe

- » **36ml lime blossom** (*Tilia cordata*). This tincture helps lighten the load, and it's specifically good for people who give out more energy than they take back for themselves.

- » **18ml rose** (*Rosa damascena*), a tincture that brings the essence of self-love into the mix that is so important when you feel everything is on you. It's important to be able to prioritise yourself too.

- » **9ml liquorice** (*Glycyrrhiza glabra*) tincture, an adaptogen that helps abate the effects of long-term stress. It will give you strength to keep going.

- » **36ml hawthorn** (*Crataegus spp.*) tincture. This is my favourite tonic, supporting the circulation and strengthening the body. It also helps with relaxation, anxiety and insomnia.

How to use
Combine and take 5ml three times a day for a month.

Let it out

- » Elecampane
- » Thyme

Got something you need to get off your chest? This is the remedy for you. This is what I'd put in my truth serum if I had one. Thyme works on the throat physically and spiritually to help you express yourself, while elecampane goes a little deeper and drags things up which you've trapped in your lungs. The lungs are traditionally seen as the place where grief is stored so show some caution before taking this remedy. You may stir up things that were better left where they were.

Recipe

- » **15ml elecampane** (*Inula helenium*), a root tincture which loosens old stuck mucous from the lungs, heats the body and unleashes whatever is trapped on the chest (emotionally and physically).

- » **15ml thyme** (*Thymus vulgaris*), a tincture which soothes a sore throat, kills any bacteria which may be causing an infection and clears the throat for you to speak freely.

How to use
Take 3 drops morning and night until you've expressed whatever it is that needed getting out.

Period cramp relief

I believe this mix works well when the period pain is mild to moderate. I found that no tincture under the sun helped relieve my pain on "the day", it was all dependent on what I'd done in the weeks preceding the pain that mattered for me. So don't feel bad if this doesn't work as "on-the-day" relief. It just means you need to put more effort into changing your lifestyle and diet instead!

Recipe

> » **30ml cramp bark** (*Viburnum opulus*), as it relieves cramps (hence the name).

> » **2ml ginger** (*Zingiber officianlis*) to improve circulation and reduce inflammation.

> » **28ml chamomile** (*Chamomilla recutita*) to relax the muscles and reduce inflammation.

How to use

Mix together and take 2ml every few hours until symptoms subside.

Herbal Monographs
[Everything they do and more]

—— *Althea officinalis* (marshmallow) ——

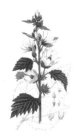

Names: mallards, mauls, schloss tea, cheeses, mortification root

Element: Water

Planet: Venus

Magical uses: psychic powers, attracts good spirits

Key words: soft, soothing, smooth, comforting, coating

Tissue state: atrophy + excitation

Qualities: cool + damp

Actions: moistening, soothing, anti-inflammatory, diuretic, emollient, demulcent, alterative, antilithic, antitussive, vulnerary

Uses: sore throat, cystitis, swollen glands, dry cough, bronchitis, asthma, emphysema, hyperacidity, ulcers, mucous colitis, low digestive enzyme production, diarrhoea, dysentry, crohns disease, constipation, haemorrhoids, hiatus hernia, gravels in urine, sore nipples, arthritis, skin inflammation, eczema, hypertension, diabetes, oedema, chemotherapy, inflamed alimentary canal, boils, abscesses, old wounds

Parts used: flowers, leaves (urinary) + roots (digestion)

Known constituents: starch, pectin, oil, sugar, asparagin, phosphate of lime, glutinois matter, cellulose, mucilage, flavonoids, tannins, salt, phenolic acids, scopoletin

Legend and tradition

In case you were wondering, marshmallow does indeed give its name to the sweet. Its roots were once used to make a rudimentary version of the marshmallow sweets we have now. The name *malvaceae* comes from the Greek word *malake*, meaning soft. The name *Althea* is from the greek *Altho*, meaning to cure (Grieves, 1992).

But before it was used as medicine it was more readily used as a food. The roots were boiled then fried with onions and butter. The trouble that they must have gone to in order to prepare this root I would assume is a reflection of how hard food was to come by rather than the deliciousness of the roots. But perhaps I should try it first.

In France, the young leaves and flowering tops are still used in salads. It's thought that the Romans probably introduced this (Grieves, 1992). But even before that, the Egyptians were recorded as eating it too. The Arab physicians would use the leaves as a poultice for inflammation and the roots as lozenges.

Medicinal uses

There are two distinct parts of this herb which are used: the roots and the leaves. There isn't much difference between the two in terms of medicinal uses so I haven't split them up in this monograph. The root is much more mucilaginous than the leaves so the roots are usually more closely associated with the digestive system, whereas the leaves are associated with the urinary system.

Digestion

I use the powdered root as an alternative to slippery elm. It coats the digestive system in a moistening layer, which protects the digestion from acids and hot foods. It also helps any trauma to the gut to heal, such as ulcers. Its anti-inflammatory action helps to reduce the heat in conditions such as crohn's and colitis (Wood, 2008).

Lungs

The root and/or leaves can be added to any cough mix to help soothe the lungs and oesophagus. It is useful in blends for asthma, emphysema and bronchitis.

Urinary

The leaves work especially well on the urinary system. Its diuretic effects will make you wee more often than usual but this is excellent in the case of a bladder infection. It's also useful when you have water retention. It will help you to clear gravel in the urine as well (Wood, 2008).

Circulatory

Its effects as a diuretic may also lower the blood pressure in some instances.

Skin

You may have heard of oats being used to make a milky bath for eczema. Marshmallow root will do something similar and is probably why it was used in the past by Arabic physicians as a poultice. To make a poultice you will want to pound up the roots and pour on boiling water. When this cools strain it through a cloth. Wrap the cold wet herb material in a clean cloth and put this on the skin. This is a cold poultice. A hot poultice would use warm herb material and usually put a hot water bottle behind it to keep it warm once it's on the body.

Safety considerations

None known

—— *Arctium lappa* (burdock) ——

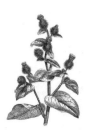

Names: lappa, fox's cote, bardana, burrseed, hurrburr, thorny burr, beggars buttons, clotbur, happy major, cockle buttons, love leaves, philanthropium, personata, appa major

Element: Water

Planet: Venus

Magical uses: wards off negativity, protection, protective necklace

Key words: deep, dark, strength, absorb, cling, clear

Tissue state: atrophy and stagnation

Qualities: oily and bitter

Actions: laxative, appetite stimulant, central nervous system stimulant, circulatory and lympathic stimulant, antifungal, diuretic, astringent, bitter tonic, antiscorbutic, relaxant, demulcent

Physical uses: dry skin, syphillis, furunculosis, eczema, psoriasis, acne, urticaria, joint disease, connective tissue disease, detoxification, blood cleansing, removes uric acid, gout, painful limbs, alopecia, balance blood sugar, stiff lower back, sciatica, carpal tunnel syndrome, profuse sweating, oedema, boils, abscess, carbuncles, arthritis, rheumatism, styes, sebhorrea, cystitis, anorexia, reduce bad cholesterol

Emotional uses: feeling worn out, emotional baggage, release toxic emotions

Parts used: root (leaves and seed also but actions above refer to root)

Known constituents: lignan, inulin (starch), mucilage, sugars, pectin, sulphur and organic acids, sesquiterpenes, tannin, iron, sulphur, B vitamins, phenolic acid, fatty acids

Legend and tradition

The latin name for burdock, *Arctium,* comes back to the Greek root, *arcos. Arcos* means "bear" and is thought to relate to the sharp claws of the burdock seeds. The velcro like hooks on these seeds catch on anything which passes it and this action lends itself to many more of its names, such as "the beggars buttons". I love the idea of someone using these to mimic buttons, though I don't think they would do a very good job! As the leaves are heart shaped I'm making a logical jump to conclude this explains its name "love leaves". While it is descriptive of its appearance it doesn't allude to any romantic uses. However, I found it interesting to see the name *Philanthropon* listed for burdock because another herb which sticks to you; cleavers, is also called this (Grieves, 1992).

Medicinal uses

The leaves were once used topically for rheumatism, gout, leprosy, kidney obstruction, venereal disease and externally on burns, scalds, and scrofulus swellings. The leaves used to be boiled in milk and used topically as a cataplasm (plaster).

Digestion and elimination

The root is bitter and oily which means that it will stimulate expulsion of metabolic waste as well as helping the body to absorb essential fatty acids, thereby moisturising the body from the inside out. This makes it useful in cases of eczema, scrofula, acne, and psoriasis. It is even useful for eczema, which causes broken and weeping skin.

I would recommend it as a bitter tonic, since it helps to increase the excretion of bile in the stomach and mucilage in the intestines.

This allows the nutrients of foods to be absorbed better. It also improves peristalsis, an integral part of absorption, as the movement of the intestines maximises the surface area of them.

The main action burdock is used for is its blood cleansing or alterative action. But what does this really mean? Blood cleansing is a bit of a misleading concept as we can't actually do this in reality. Some describe it as; "medicines that alter the process of nutrition, restoring in some unknown way the normal functions of an organ or system... re. establishing healthy nutritive process" – *Blakiston's Medical dictionary.*

By increasing bile, sweat and urine it helps us eliminate metabolic waste from the system. It is thought that this enables burdock to flush uric acid from the body and improve joint pains caused by rheumatism, arthritis and gout.

Skin

I love to use burdock in my dispensary and it usually makes an appearance when I need to treat a skin condition which causes dryness and dehydration. This is probably what most herbalists think of burdock as for. It is the root that is normally used in modern practice.

Urinary

Burdock is excellent for helping to clear swollen feet or hands. This is because it has a diuretic action. In fact, the seeds were traditionally used to help move fluids and are stronger in their diuretic action than the root.

Immunity

Another type of swelling burdock helps is when the lymphatic system is inflamed while trying to deal with an infection.

Reproduction

Matthew Wood connects the burdock's ability to absorb and utilise fats as essential to the movement of hormones in the body. He sees it as a potentially very helpful remedy in the support of hormonal balance for women. This would be best suited for women who are menstruating or premenopausal as it is normally not recommended to use herbs which have sesquiterpenes during pregnancy. However, having said that, I did find reference to it being used during pregnancy in the past to nourish the mother.

I personally wouldn't recommend using burdock for nourishment during pregnancy without seeing a herbalist.

Safety considerations

Asteracea allergy. Shouldn't be used during pregnancy, breast-feeding, when taking lithium or diuretic drugs.

—— Avena sativa (oat) ——

Names: groats, oatmeal

Element: Earth

Planet: Venus

Magical uses: blessing the harvest, money, fertility, endurance, inner peace

Key words: soothe, build up, nourish, calm

Tissue state: atrophy, excitation

Qualities: moistening

Actions: nervine, antidepressant, tranquiliser, brain tonic, cardiac tonic, thymoleptic, antispasmodic

Physical uses: adrenal fatigue, depression, anxiety, debility, neurasthenia, tension, irritability, insomnia, shingles, hyperactive kids, tremor, Parkinson's, low libido, tachycardia, palpitations, PMS, headaches, exhaustion, shoulder tension

Emotional uses: despondency, apathy, "spaceyness"

Parts used: flowering tops and straw

Known constituents: glycosyl flavones, proteins, Vitamin E, proteins, iron, zinc, manganese

Legend and tradition

Oats have been an important part of British farming for quite some time. It is believed that the oats should be left for the church bells to ring three times before they are brought inside after harvest. This essentially gave a 3-week time period for them to dry in the sun

Medicinal uses

Oat tops are one of my favourite tonics for building up someone's energy. I use it for people who feel tired and wired. I once made a blend of elderflower and oat tops for a student who was clearly on edge but said she didn't understand why she wasn't able to sleep. This gentle nudge was all she needed to sleep better and feel energized again during the day. What's especially nice about oat tops is that they don't overstimulate as some of the adaptogens do. It's a good starting point for anyone with adrenal fatigue, depression, or anxiety. I think of it as bubble wrap for the nerves. Coating them in a protective layer when the nerves are agitated and frayed.

Circulation

It is sometimes used for tachycardia and palpitations. Not because it has a direct effect upon the cardiovascular system but because it supports the nerves and reduces their excitation, which would lead to such circulation problems.

Reproductive

It shouldn't come as a surprise that oat tops help with PMS. I like to think of PMS as a highlighting of whatever is already happening in your life. It's not a hormone imbalance and it very rarely needs hormonal herbs. When we assume a hormone is to blame we're partaking of the thought process that women, and their hormones, make them a bit hysterical. It's better to own these feelings rather than brush them off. Oat tops allows us to lessen our sensitivity to outside environment and allows us to take a calmer approach to whatever may be bothering us.

Safety considerations

If you have coeliac disease or severe gluten intolerance it's best to avoid this herb, but most oat top suppliers don't grow their plants next to or after wheat so there shouldn't really be any gluten in it. But best avoided to be on the safe side.

—— *Calendula officinalis* (marigold) ——

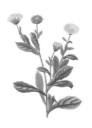

Names: *Calendula officinalis* (Latin) marybud, marigold, gold-bloom, Summer's bride, husbandman's dial, holigold, Bride of the Sun, spousa solis, golds, gold, golds, the sun's gold, ball's eyes, bees-love, oculis-christi, drunkard, marygold, mary gowles, ruddles, ruddes, solis sponsa, solsequia

Element: Fire

Planet: Sun

Magical uses: protection, divination, find lost items, prevent or stop gossip, happiness and joy

Tissue type: depression

Qualities: warming +

Actions: immune stimulant, antiprotozoal, anti-inflammatory, antifungal, antispasmodic, anti-haemorrhage, antihistamine, antibacterial, active against staphylococcus and streptococcus, antiemetic, anticancer, antiseptic, styptic, haemostatic, diaphoretic, anthelmintic, oetrogenic activity, menstrual regulator

Physical uses: eczema, wound healing, lacerations, grazes, ulcers, abscesses, sore nipples, stop bleeding, varicose veins, chilblains, fistulas, radiotherapy burns, thrush, sunburn, insect bites, bruises, infection, colitis, balanitis, gallbladder inflammation, endometriosis, infertility, amenorrhea, painful periods, leucorrhea, irritated vaginal walls, tearing in childbirth (externally), heavy periods, hot flushes, fibroids

Emotional uses: uplifting, antidepressant, grief

Parts used: flowers

Constituents: triterpenes; pentacyclic alcohols; flavonoids including rutin; resins; saponins; sesquiterpene glycosides; volatile oils and polysaccharides; bitters, phytosterols, mucilage, carotenoids such as carotene and calendulin

Legend and tradition

In the language of flowers it would be used to symbolise grief. When combined with roses it could represent the bittersweet pains of love. This association with death in Europe is mirrored in Mexico where it is used as decoration on the day of the dead (Grieves, 1992).

Skin

Marigold is well known for its external uses as it is often found in creams to help heal the skin. It is known to help heal dry skin in eczema but it can also be used to heal wounds including ulcers.

It can be used as a cream on sore nipples as this will prevent the transferral of thrush at the same time.

Marigold is less commonly known for its internal uses although it has many obvious applications once you know the external uses. For instance, just as it is used on ulcers externally it can be used internally, such as when treating stomach ulcers. It can also be used to treat thrush in the throat and vagina, as well as on the skin, as previously mentioned.

Immune
As a lymphatic it is useful in reducing inflammation in the system (including immune hyperactivity). It is helpful in reducing raised glands in common colds and will break a fever in flu. As an anti-inflammatory it is used to treat colitis, balanitis and gallbladder inflammation.

Liver
It is a mild bitter and will help digestion but it is also known for treating jaundice.

Reproductive
It is said by Matthew Wood to increase the life force in the pelvic region. As such it can be used for myriad problems. These include endometriosis, infertility, amenorrhea, painful periods, leucorrhoea, irritated vaginal walls, tearing in childbirth (externally), heavy periods and hot flushes and fibroids in the menopause.

Safety considerations
None known.

— *Capsella bursa-pastoris* (shepherd's purse) —

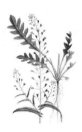

Names: shepherd's bag, shepherd's scrip, shepherd's sprout, lady's purse, witches pouch, rattle pouches, cese-weed, pick-pocket, pick-purse, bindweed, pepper and salt, poor man's parmacettie, sanginary, mother's heart, Diana's heart, Diana's arrow head, clappedepouch

Element: Earth

Planet: Saturn

Magical uses: divination, hecate

Key words: stop, strengthening, "no", boundaries

Tissue state: depression + excitation

Qualities: cold + dry

Actions: haemostatic, urinary antiseptic, diuretic, astringent, hypotensive, emmenagogue, antiuric acid, circulatory stimulant

Physical uses: blood in urine, menorrhagia, leucorrhea, puss in urine, irritable bowel, vomitting blood, nosebleeds, diarrhoea, thrush, fibroids, endometriosis, cystitis, dysentry, bedwetting, kidney stones, bladder stones, intermittent fever

Emotional uses: for empaths, easily overwhelmed by their senses, will tone the energetic body

Parts used: aerial parts

Known constituents: histamine, tyramine, flavonoids, plant acids, resins, volatile oils, organic acid, carotenoids, vitamins A, K, and C, potassium, amino acids

Legend and tradition

The names shepherd's purse, witches pouch and lady's purse, are in reference to the old leather purses of shepherd's which had a similar shape to the seed pods. Sometimes it is also associated with the Goddess Diana as the seed pods are likened to her arrow heads.

The Irish name "clappedepouch" refers to a time when lepers would beg at the corners of streets using a clapper or bell and receive alms at the end of a pole (Grieves, 1992).

Legend has it that the plant helps relieve jaundice when bound to the soles of the feet. Though I have not found any modern reference confirming this.

Medicinal uses

Reproductive

As with most herbs, shepherd's purse is best known for one thing. In this case, its ability to stop heavy periods. I have used it for young girls who have just started menstruating and women who are losing lots of blood in menopause. I don't know that it has a specific effect on the hormones but rather helps through its haemostatic action on the blood itself.

It's astringent properties are so strong that it can help to tone the uterus enough to heal if it is atrophied.

Circulation

It might come as a surprise, then, to learn that this herb is also a circulatory stimulant. How paradoxical that it can stop blood and move it too. This is just a wonderful example of the balancing properties so many herbs have.

Digestion

It is not uncommon that the tissue state which causes illness in the vagina also impacts upon the digestive and urinary systems as these sit right next to each other. I have had patients who suffered with recurring urinary infections and who, once these were repaired, were suddenly able to conceive. Yet this connection is not acknowledged in modern medicine. By using a herb such as shepherd's purse to tone the uterus you are also toning the digestive system.

When the digestive system does not have *enough* tone it struggles to absorb and break down food correctly. This can lead to conditions of diarrhoea and irritable bowel.

Urinary

Shepherd's purse is great for toning the bladder too, where it helps to treat cystitis and bedwetting (Wood, 2008).

Safety considerations

Do not use during pregnancy, and have caution with those who have hypothyroidism (Wood, 2008).

—— *Chamomilla recutita* (chamomile) ——

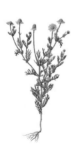

Names: *Chamomilla recutita, Matricaria recutita* or *Matricaric chamomilla*, manzanilla

Element: Fire

Planet: Sun

Magical uses: money, sleep, love, purification, increase passion, empower young girls, hung above cribs for strength

Key words: gentle, childlike, playful, cheerful, strong

Tissue state: irritation, constriction and stagnation

Qualities: hot and dry

Actions: anti-inflammatory, antimicrobial, antiseptic, anti-peptic ulcer, anodyne, antispasmodic, bitter tonic, carminative, vulnerary, mild nerve sedative, antihistamine, analgesic, decongestant, relaxant

Physical uses: colic, tension, IBS, constipation, diarrhoea, gastritis, ulcers, Crohn's disease, nausea, motion sickness, fever, diverticulitis, colitis, sore throats, sinusitis, coughs, cystitis, heartburn, nausea during pregnancy, painful periods, delayed menses, hot flushes, mastitis, premenstrual head-aches, migraines, neuralgia, carpal tunnel syndrome, toothache, teething, earache, cramp, rheumatism, gout, eczema, psoriasis, hay fever, asthma, wounds, ulcers, urticaria, cysts, sores, burns, scalds, impetigo, blisters, sore nipples, eye infection and conjunctivitis (pink eye)

Emotional uses: mental tension, for people who whine about things, suitable for babies of all ages, prickly oversensitive volatile people

Parts used: aerial parts

Known constituents: volatile oils, flavonoids, coumarins, plant acids, fatty acids, cyanogenic glycosides, salicylate derivatives, choline and tannin

Legend and tradition

The word chamomile comes from the Greek *khamaemelon* meaning "earth apple". This is due to it's fruity fragrance. In the language of flowers chamomile means patience or energy in adversity. This is because it derives strength from being trodden on (Grieves, 1992).

Medicinal uses

Bitter tastes are crucial to the digestive system. They encourage the intestines to contract and relax in waves, called peristalsis, and they help us create bile in preparation for breaking down foods in the stomach. Chamomile will aid in both constipation and diarrhoea and is often used in IBS for this reason.

Nerves

The connection from the gut to the mind is incredible and this is sometimes strongest in children. They communicate through their tummies and bowels. Even low level stress may cause chronic constipation. Chamomile is great for this.

Digestion

Chamomile is also prebiotic, helping to balance the bowel flora which is upset by IBS. It can be used to relieve gastritis, ulcers, Crohn's disease, colic in infants and other digestive problems.

A strong infusion will bring out the bitter properties of the herb and makes a good aperitif 30 mins before a meal. It is this preparation that also has an emmenagogue effect. This means it will help bring on a period and potentially a miscarriage in early stages of pregnancy. Chamomile is otherwise perfectly safe to drink through pregnancy, just don't infuse it for over 5 minutes, to be on the safe side. Grieves says the strong infusions can be emetic (make you vomit), though I've never experienced this.

Immune

As an antiseptic it is useful against colds and flus but especially useful for thrush in women. It helps alleviate fever, sore throat, sinusitis, coughs and cystitis. A worthy herb for first aid in every home.

Reproductive

The relaxing effects help to relieve nausea during pregnancy and uterine contractions in painful periods. It is a very gentle emmenagogue and very useful when menses is delayed due to stress. It reduces menopausal symptoms where stress is a major contributor to hot symptoms. It also relieves mastitis, premenstrual headaches and migraines.

Immune

Its antihistamine action makes it useful in treating eczema, asthma and hay fever.

Skin

It's also great for wounds, ulcers, sores, burns, sore nipples and scalds when applied in a cream or poultice. Another way to use it externally is in the form of a douche for cystitis and thrush and as an eyewash for eye infections, inflammation or irritations.

Safety considerations

Avoid long infusions of the herb during the first trimester of pregnancy.

—— *Cinnamomum zeylanicum* (cinnamon) ——

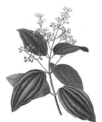

Names: blume, *Laurus cinnamomum*

Element: Fire

Planet: Sun

Magical uses: love spells, good luck, temple purification, mental focus and divination

Key words: warm

Tissue state: depression, atrophy and relaxation

Qualities: warming, stimulating, astringent

Actions: stimulant astringent, antispasmodic, haemostatic, antiseptic, vermifuge, aromatic, antimicrobial, carminative

Physical uses: hypoglycaemia, diabetes, PCOS, heavy periods, rheumatism, sore muscles, fever with chills, colds, flu, congestion, parasites, low appetite, flatulence, nausea, diarrhoea, griping, IBS, bronchitis

Emotional uses: depression, frigidity

Parts used: bark from the shoots

Known constituents: tannins, mucilage, essential oils, coumarin

Caution: Don't use in medicinal doses in pregnancy (cooking with the spice is perfectly safe)

Legend and tradition

Cinnamon has been used for medicine and magic for centuries. The cassia variety originates from China and was imported to Egypt as early as 2000 BC, where it was used in the mummification of the dead. The cinnamon we use in cooking, and referred to in this monograph, comes from India where the herb was heavily protected so that its whereabouts was unknown to most, thereby ensuring it could not be stolen (Grieves, 1992).

Medicinal uses

The gentle warming effect of cinnamon makes it a wonderful addition to any hot toddy when you have a cold or flu, are feeling congested or have a fever with chills.

Musculoskeletal

It also helps warm the muscles and joints to aid with soreness and rheumatism. Rheumatism is usually made worse by cold wet weather so warming the body from the inside can really help.

Digestion

Cinnamon is antiparasitic and can be used for the pinworms and tapeworms that are common during childhood. As with most spices it helps to abate flatulence, colic, and IBS.

Endocrine

Cinnamon has a balancing effect on the blood sugar that makes it useful in diabetes and the insulin resistance that often leads to (or accompanies) PCOS. It can also be used to lessen a heavy period.

Safety considerations

None known.

—— *Citrus aurantium flos* (orange blossom) ——

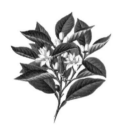

Names: bigardier, seville orange, bitter orange, vitrus dulcis

Element: Fire

Planet: Neptune

Magical uses: strength to any seeker or adventurer, romance and fertility

Key words: uplift, happiness, cheer, magical messenger

Tissue state: depressed

Qualities: relaxing, stimulating, possible aphrodisiac

Actions: anti-inflamatory

Physical uses: mastitis, leucorrhea, rheumatism, arthristis, upper respiratory infections, cough

Emotional uses: find your flow, ease grief

Parts used: flower

Known constituents: volatile oil

Legend and tradition

Citrus aurantium makes a few essential oils from its different parts. The flower makes neroli, the leaves and young shoots make petit-grain and the fruit skin makes orange oil. Neroli is extremely expensive, as so much of the plant is required to make it. It also takes a lot of time and farming space to be usable. Bergamot, which is made from a slightly different citrus, is easier to come by and smells similar to neroli, so is often used as an alternative. I love the abundance of smells found in one plant (Grieves, 1992).

Medicinal uses

Nervous

Orange blossom is one of my most used herbs. The irony is that I don't really know what it does physically. I only ever use it in small doses for emotional reasons instead. I was taught at university that it acts as a carrier for your intentions and makes sure the medicine goes where it needs to. Literally, a touch of magic.

Aside from the magical uses I employ it has a wonderfully uplifting, antidepressing effect. It just helps people move up and out of their problems. I love it dearly.

Immunity

It supports the immune system, especially the upper respiratory tract when it is inflamed. This is the area of the body that many people store grief and I would certainly think this herb useful for such a situation.

Reproductive

The ability for this herb to help you find flow and movement in the body enables it in relieving a late period or a painful one. Its anti-inflammatory properties make it useful in mastitis. Though I don't see an obvious physiological reason why, it might help with leucorrhea (a bacterial imbalance in the vagina).

Musculoskeletal
This herb also helps you move physically, reducing inflammation in the joints and aiding rheumatism.

Safety considerations
None known

—— *Crataegus laevigata* (hawthorn) ——

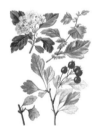

Names: may, bread and cheese, hagthorn, moon flower, whitethorn, quickthorn, may tree, mayblossom, ladies' meat, gaxels, halves, huath, may bush, mayflower, tree of chastity and quickset. The berries are known as haws, chucky cheese, cuckoo's beads and pixie pears

Element: Fire

Planet: Mars

Magical uses: associated with fairies and Blodeuwedd. The berries can be used in magic to encourage more dynamism, courage, clarity and insight in your life. It will also help develop initiative

Key words: heart, love, relax, strengthen, repair, dynamic

Tissue type: excitation, atrophy and relaxation

Qualities: cool and dry

Actions: cardiotonic, cardiac, diuretic, astringent, relaxant, antioxidant, antispasmodic

Physical uses: hypertension and hypotension, hypercholesterolaemia, strengthens the heart muscles, myocarditis, arteriosclerosis, atheroma, thrombosis, paroxysmal tachycardia, angina, enlargement of the heart from overwork, dizziness, intermittent claudication, insomnia, anxiety, overexertion and mental tension, kidney stones, inflammation of the mucosa, memory enhancer, palpitations, menopause, draws out thorns and splinters, heart failure, cystitis and sore throat

Emotional uses: mend a broken heart, open the heart chakra, unblock problems receiving and giving love, softens anger, anxiety, restlessness, irritability, nervousness

Parts used: leaf, flower and berry

Known constituents: bioflavanoids, triterpenoids, proanthocyanins, coumarins, amines, ascorbic acid (in berries only) and saponins (in the berries only)

Legend and tradition

It is used in May Queen rituals and would often be worn in the hair by the May Queen. Its smell is likened to the smell of a woman's sexual organs when aroused. As such it is associated with fertility, just as May Day is.

It is said that the flowers encourage fairies to come into the house. It is for this reason that it is thought by some to be lucky and by others unlucky to bring into the home. It is also said to be unlucky to pick the blossom before May, but this can't be helped if this is what weather brings about, as the blossom doesn't last long on the trees (Grieves, 1992).

Medicinal uses

Cardiovascular

Hawthorn is well know for its association with the heart. It helps to open (dilate) arteries but also helps strengthen the heart muscle. This combination of actions gives it the ability to strengthen those with low blood pressure and those with high blood pressure alike. Not only does it dilate the blood vessels but it also helps to clear dangerous cholesterol (LDL), it protects against plaque forming in the arteries preventing and treating heart attack, angina and arrhythmias.

Digestion

In Chinese medicine the berries are used to help strengthen the digestive powers for eating meat as it helps the absorption of animal fats. In fact, it is often cooked alongside meat in that part of the world. The berry can be used in medicine to help moisten the gut walls and aid effective absorption. It may be useful in leaky gut syndrome for this reason but I have yet to test this theory.

Nerves

Hawthorn can also be used to lower anxiety levels. It can also be used to relieve insomnia. Because of its cooling and calming properties it is used by some herbalists to help alleviate the hyperactivity of those with ADD and ADHD.

Immune

Its cooling effects also make it useful in inflammation such as rheumatism, arthritis and other autoimmune problems. Eczema, hayfever, sinusitis and asthma may all benefit from hawthorn as they generally come about from a hot and excited tissue state. It could be likened to an antihistamine although it doesn't act through the histamine constituent.

Safety considerations

There are no known potential safety problems with this herb.

—— *Galium aperine* (cleavers) ——

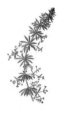

Names: *Galium aperine* in Latin. Sometimes called goosegrass, borweed, hedgeriff, hayriffe, eriffe, grip grass, hayruff, catchweed, scratweed, mutton chops, Robin-run-in-the-grass, love-man, goosebill, everlasting-friendship, clite, click, clitheren, clithers, philanthropen, sticky-willy, cleaverwort, bedstraw

Element: Water

Planet: Moon

Magical uses: relationships, commitment, protection, tenacity

Key words: stretch, grab, cling, scratch, climb

Tissue state: dry or atrophic

Qualities: cool and moist

Actions: lymphatic alterative and detoxifier, diuretic, astringent tonic, anti-inflammatory, antiobesity, adaptogen and antineoplastic

Physical uses: skin ailments, clearing the lymph, cystitis, urethritis, prostatitis, orchitis, chickenpox, measles, traditionally used in labour as deer use it as such, nodular goitre, obesity, psoriasis, eruptions, boils, eczema, bedwetting, acne, blood cleanser, cancers, cysts, fibroids, catarrh, lymph swelling, insomnia, dupuytren's contracture, morton's neuroma, fatigue, especially during labour

Emotional uses: nervous excess, brings inner calm, peace and tranquility

Parts used: aerial parts

Known constituents: anthraquinone derivatives, flavonoids, iridoids, polyphonic acids

Legend and tradition

Many of the names of cleaver's originate from the anglo-saxon "hedge-riff" meaning tax gatherer or robber. This refers to its ability to pluck wool from sheep as they pass by. Its latin name *aperine* comes from the Greek aparo meaning "to seize". "Clite", "click", "clitheren" and "clithers" are all forms of the word "cleavers". Cleaver's coming from "to cleave", meaning "stick fast to", "adhere strongly", and "become very strongly involved with or emotionally attached to someone" (Grieves, 1992).

Its other names, "everlasting friendship" or "love-man" seems to come from this meaning.

Medicinal uses

Immunity

This plant has a traditional association with the immune system as a "blood cleanser". This is an old term used for substances which would help to clear infection by way of the lymphatic system before we knew much about anatomy and physiology. As such it is useful in fevers, eruptions, boils, abscesses, dermatitis, eczema, scrofula, "pocks of the skin" and teen acne.

Urinary

Its ability to combat infection is especially strong in the urinary system as it is a diuretic. As such it is useful against cystitis, prostatitis, urethritis, gall stones, orchitis, and soreness of the testes.

Nerves

It's very helpful for nervousness, excitability and insomnia and was once used in epilepsy.

Safety Considerations

None known

—— *Glycyrrhiza glabra* (liquorice) ——

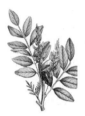

Names: sweet root, *Liquiritia officinalis*, Lycorys

Element: air

Planet: mercury

Magical uses: lust, love, and fidelity

Key words: sweet, strength, energy

Tissue state: atrophy, depression

Qualities: warming, moistening, stimulating

Actions: demulcent, expectorant, glycogen-conserver, anti-inflammatory, mild laxative, adaptogen, oestrogenic, antiulcer, antiviral, antidepressive, antidiuretic, antihistamine, antioxidant

Physical uses: adrenal fatigue, addison's disease, hypoglycaemia, peptic ulcer, IBS, Crohn's, mouth ulcer, dry cough, hoarseness, tuberculosis, catarrh, bronchitis, urinary tract infection

Emotional uses: passions, sexual healing, frozen or afraid of these emotions.

Parts used: root

Known constituents: volatile oil, coumarins, chalcones, triterpenes, flavonoids

Legend and tradition

Many people who grew up in World War Two will remember liquorice, as it was grown in the UK to be sold as a sweet when sugar was hard to come by. Its latin name is very descriptive of the plant, *glukos* meaning sweet and *riza* meaning root. It is said you can survive 10 days without food or water so long as you have liquorice root to chew on. Although it originates from South-East Europe and South-West Asia it can, and has, been grown in the UK for a long time (Grieves, 1992).

Medicinal Uses

Digestion – Liquorice isn't just sweet; it also coats whatever it touches in a soothing layer. This is known as being demulcent. It helps peptic ulcers to heal, as well as Crohn's diease and mouth ulcers.

Endocrine

The herb is most often used as an adaptogen, helping to support the adrenal glands when they have been in overdrive for a long time. It can have a steroidal-like effect on the body and makes it useful in Addison's disease.

Respiratory

The lovely soothing effect of liquorice is most obviously felt on the tongue and throat when you drink the tea. It has been tradi-tionally used in cough syrups for hundreds of years as a result.

Safety Considerations

Shouldn't be used if you have high blood pressure or liver cirrhosis and is to be avoided during pregnancy in case it raises blood pressure.

—— *Hyssopus officianlis* (hyssop) ——

Names: hyssop, hyssopus

Element: Air

Planet: Jupiter

Magical uses: cleansing, purification, repels negative energy, protects house from intruders, protects healers from contracting the illness of the patient

Key words: clearing, moving, uplifting, cleansing

Tissue state: depression

Qualities: warm, diffusive

Actions: pyretic, expectorant, emmenagogue, mild analgesics, diuretic, antispasmodic, external antispasmodic, antiviral (herpes simplex)

Physical uses: bronchitis, sore throat, colds, chills, catarrh, nervous asthma, sinusitis, increased appetite, hysteria, urinary infection, cold sores

Emotional uses: phobia, guilt, compulsions, obsession, drowning in feeling

Parts used: leaves

Known constituents: volatile oils, flavonoids, terpenoids, mucilage, resin

Legend and tradition

The name hyssop comes from *azob* meaning "Holy" in Greek. Hyssop has been associated with religion for centuries. It was used to purify the air and energy of a place and is still used to consecrate Westminster Abbey (Grieves, 1992).

Medicinal Uses

Respiratory – I'd say I mostly associate hyssop with the respiratory system. I often see it as a gentler version of thyme. It is antiviral so should be thought of as your first line of defense against a cold. It helps alleviate catarrh, sinusitis, constrictive coughs and even nervous asthma.

The trouble with nervous asthma is that the nervous system is being stimulated into constricting. What's nice about hyssop is that it helps open the bronchioles by relaxing the spasm. This leads me to believe the herb must have some effect on the nervous system as well.

Immunity

The antiviral properties of this plant make it a wonderful alternative or complement to thyme. They are closely related and work well together. Like thyme, it treats colds and chills. It has even been shown to have effects against *herpes simplex* (cold sores).

Digestion

The warmth of hyssop makes it a gentle herb to improve digestion.

Safety Considerations

None known

—— *Inula helenium* (elecampane) ——

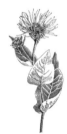

Names: elfwort, elf dock, horseheal, nurseheal, scabwort, velvet dock, wild sunflower

Element: Air

Planet: Mercury

Magical uses: love, protection, psychic powers

Key words: hot, exciting, energy, oomph, kapow!

Tissue state: depression, stagnation and atrophy

Qualities: hot + dry

Actions: antispasmodic, alterative, stimulating expectorant, diaphoretic, antiseptic, stomachic, anticatarrhal, antibacterial

Physical uses: old coughs, tuberculosis, haemoptysis, whooping cough, croup, cough up, old phlegm, silicosis, pneumoconiosis, emphysema, chronic catarrh, night sweats, leucorrhea, strengthen digestion, stitches in the side, hyperventilation, asthma, detoxing, depression, poor concentration, hoarseness, diphtheria, postnasal drip, shallow breath, loss of appetite, gastric atonicity, wind and spasm, rheumatic pain, cramps, convulsions, paralysis, fever, snake bite

Emotional uses: enables the embodiment, bringing someone who exists in their head into their body

Parts used: root

Known constituents: sesquiterpene lactones, inulin, resin, helenin, volatile oils, bitters, triterpenes, mucilage, resin, sterols

Legend and tradition

The name helenium is said to come from the name Helen, as in Helen of Troy. A story goes that she cried when Paris took her away, and that where her tears fell the elecampane grew (Grieves, 1992).

Its names elfshot and elfwort comes from the belief that it could be used to treat wasting and preoccupation caused by being shot by an elfin arrowhead (Wood, 2008).

Medicinal Uses

Lungs

The pungent taste of the elecampane makes it excellent for punching through the stickiness of old phlegm. It is particularly indicated when the phlegm is green as this is a sign of infection. Elecampane is antibacterial and will help to thin it as well as changing its colour.

Asthma is the most common cause of shortness of breath. Elecampane is likely to be helpful because it helps to break down mucous. But it is possible that it also relaxes the bronchioles.

Digestion

Strengthens the body by improving loss of appetite, elecampane will sustain the spirit.

Reproduction

The antibacterial properties of elecampane don't just apply to the lungs though. It is also useful for leucorrhea. This is an unusual discharge for the vagina that can be perfectly normal without any underlying problem. But it can also be caused by bacterial infection. I found it immensely curious to hear the other day of a myth regarding fertility. Apparently, sometimes in the USA, doctors recommend drinking cough syrup during ovulation to help with implantation of a fertilised egg by thinning the vaginal mucous. But, it doesn't work like that, it's specifically works on thinning the mucous in the lungs and I couldn't find any reason why that action would also work on the vaginal mucous, as they're not being produced by the same processes. However, here we are, talking about how elecampane works on changing the quality of the vaginal mucous in the instance where bacteria is the cause. I still think the cough medicine wouldn't work. But I do wonder, is this thought process on the doctors behalf a reflection of how we used to use herbs??

Nerves

The strength of spirit that elecampane imbibes also helps to lift depression and helps you stay focussed too. It is especially good when there is a nervous element to a cough.

Immunity

Its strengthening, fiery nature that gives your spirit strength also strengthens your immunity.

Safety considerations

Do not use during pregnancy or lactation. Avoid in sanguine and choleric people.

—— *Medicago sativa* (alfalfa) ——

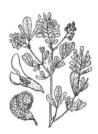

Names: purple medick, lucerne, california clover, buffalo herb

Element: Earth

Planet: Jupiter

Magical uses: protection, attracts money, protects against financial loss

Key words: grounding, strengthening

Tissue state: atrophy or torpor

Qualities: sweet, earthen, cooling

Actions: anti cholesterol, anti-haemorrhagic, anti-anaemia, anticoagulant, anti-diabetic

Physical uses: insomnia, itchy scalp, hayfever, allergies, sinusitis, sore throat, poor appetite, tooth decay, strong bones, osteopaenia, improve weight, vitality, hyperlipidaemia, bloating, abdominal pain, peptic ulcer, flatulence, rectal itching, diverticulosis, colitis, fistula, dyspepsia, cystitis, urethritis, prostatis, arthritis, gout, muscle cramp, stiffness, bruising, anaemia, lumbago, water retention, gravel, morning sickness, lactation

Emotional uses: nervousness, and irritability

Parts used: leaf

Known constituents: alkaloids, isoflavones, coumarins, sterols, amylase, coagulase, invertase, emulsin, peroxidase, lipase, pectinase, protase, vitamins A, B2, B3, B6, B12, C, D, K, P and U. Calcium, potassium, iron and phosphorous

Legend and tradition
Alfalfa is a clover native to central Asia and one of the oldest

cultiavated plants. Its name comes from the Arabic *al-fac-facah*, which means "father of all foods". Once used as a source of protein for livestock, it is now popular to sprout the plant and serve it on salads (Wood, 2008).

Medicinal uses

Immunity

Rich in vitamins and minerals, this herb builds the body up from the inside out. This strengthens immunity and lowers hyperactive reactions like hayfever and allergies. It has a soothing, nourishing taste that may remind you of drinking a comforting soup when you're sick, excellent for the inflammation of a sore throat or sinusitis.

Musculoskeletal

It is said that alfalafa can help strengthen the bones, perhaps even abating tooth decay! It is certainly worth thinking of for premenopausal ladies to strengthen their bones, or anyone who has low oestrogen for that matter as oestrogen has a clever role to play in strengthening bones.

Digestion

As with most strengthening herbs, it supports digestion. After all, our food is where we derive all our strength. Alfalfa helps to improve weight and vitality, makes sure you reduce your bad cholesterol and helps with digestive complaints such as bloating, pain, flatulence and even the inflammatory disease colitis.

Reproductive

During pregnancy it is safe to drink this herb and I almost always include it in a tea I make for the last trimester. Nourishing the body in this way always helps with breast milk supply, and it even helps with morning sickness.

Urinary

As a diuretic it helps you to flush bacteria out of the bladder. Although it isn't antibacterial, drinking lots of an anti-inflammatory herb that helps you pee frequently can sometimes be all you need.

Safety considerations

None known

—— *Melissa officinalis* (lemonbalm) ——

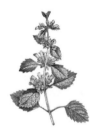

Names: sweet balm, balm, bee balm, lemon balsam, sweet melissa, oghoul, tourengane

Element: Water

Planet: Moon (Scott Cunningham), Jupiter (Culpeper)

Magical uses: love, luck, past life regression

Key words: lemon, light, bright, yellow

Tissue state: constriction

Qualities: cool + sedating

Actions: antispasmodic, antidepressant, antihistamine, antiviral, antistress, antiflatulent, febrifuge, mild tranquiliser, nerve relaxant, heart sedating, carminative, diaphoretic

Physical uses: hyperthyroidism and hypothyroidism, dizziness, migraine, nervous heart or stomach, nervousness, depression, panic attacks, nervous headache, dyspepsia, flatulence, insomnia, little energy, stomach cramps, urinary infection, feverishness, mumps, shingles, reaction to vaccination or innoculation, nervous excitability, strengthens resistance to shock and stress, low spirits, restlessness, fidgety limbs, cold and miserable, anxiety and neurosis, cleanses sores, gout pain, hyperadrenalism, palpitations, atrial fibrilation, hypertension, aneurysm, sweaty palms, fertility, menorrhagia, leucorrhea, hot flushes,impotence, blisters, herpes, stings and burns

Emotional uses: shock, mild depression, postnatal depression, lifts you out of the dark and into the light

Parts used: aerial parts, mostly leaf

Known constituents: flavonoids, triterpenes and volatile oils

Legend and tradition

It is rare that the name of a plant is used to describe the scent of a plant, but this is the case with lemonbalm. In Greek the name means bee. It is also sometimes called "beebalm", as the smell attracts bees and is favoured by them (Hughes and Owen, 2016).

Medicinal uses

Nerves

lemonbalm is probably the primary antidepressant in my dispensary, rather than St. John's Wort. But most tinctures I taste of the herb don't really capture this action. When it is macerated for too long it has more of a nourishing taste, like nettle, and loses the precious essential oils which give it its uplifting properties. The fresh herb is, of course, the best for this. It seems in the past that fresh herb preserved in wines was common.

Not only is lemonbalm good for depression, it's also useful for anxiety. Paracelsus says it's revivifying, and good for all states preceded by a disordered nervous system. I would specify that it's especially good where the nervous system is hyperactive (or "excited", to speak traditionally). I would use it for nervousness, panic attacks, nervous headache, nervous excitability, restlessness, fidgety limbs, and hyperthyroidism (Brooke, 1992).

Cardiovascular

Lemonbalm also has an affinity for the cardiovascular system, helping with aneurysm, palpitations and atrial fibrilation. Wood says it is indicated in those with sweaty palms (Wood, 2008).

Skin

Pliny and Gerard said it helps wounds to heal, the oils are so high in hydrocarbons they contain so little oxygen that the atomic germs of disease are starved out (Grieves, 1992).

Digestion

Recently, a great herbalist died: Christopher Hedley. I had the pleasure of attending only one of his talks, but he taught a whole generation of herbalists. He was an inspirational, fairy wisp of a man. He told me that sour tastes complement bitter. Both of which aid the digestion. Lemonbalm certainly fits that criteria. It is a sour plant which helps the digestion by calming it. Culpeper said that it helped digestion and brain obstructions. I love that Culpeper did not see the two organs as totally unrelated to one another as modern medicine has for so long (Culpeper, 1653).

Immunity

As a febrifuge, lemonbalm helps to sweat off a fever. It can be given as a tea for mumps, shingles and reactions to vaccination/inoculation. It won't kill all viruses but it will help break a fever, whatever the cause (Wood, 2008).

Reproductive

I hadn't used lemonbalm for sexual health before, but was pleasantly surprised to find it useful for painful periods and leucorrhea. Unsurprisingly, it also aids with hot flushes. The relaxing action and cardiovascular support it gives helps with male impotence and fertility too. Perhaps most fascinating of all is its use for retained placenta by Culpeper. Something rightfully aided by emergency intervention nowadays (Culpeper, 1653).

Safety Considerations
Not safe in pregnancy but fine for lactation. Some think it's contraindicated in hypothyroidism, others don't.

—— *Mentha piperita* (peppermint) ——

Names: brandy mint, mint

Element: Fire

Planet: Mercury

Magical uses: attract money, purification, sleep, love, psychic powers

Key words: pow! heady, pungent, stomach, cool, fresh

Tissue state: constriction and depression

Qualities: warming then cooling, stimulating

Actions: digestive, carminative, antispasmodic, diaphoretic, antiemetic, mild sedative, emmenagogue, peripheral vasodilator, enzyme activator, nervine, analgesic. aromatic stimulant, sudorific

Physical uses: Crohn's disease, diverticula, travel sickness, nausea, flatulence, anorexia (lack of appetite), cramps, spasm, muscular pain, low backache, sports injuries, stiffness, insect repellant, colds and fever, headaches, mouth sores, sore throat, heartburn, belching, hiccups, gallbladder colic, griping pains, menstrual cramps, indigestion, morning sickness, mastitis, hot or dry joints, shingles, herpes, hysteria, dizziness, fainting

Emotional uses: balances excess melancholy, strengthens expression of emotion, helps those with a sense of sadness, nervous and faint-hearted people

Parts used: leaves

Known constituents: flavonoids, acetic acid, tannins, resins, gum, triterpenes, essential oils

Legend and tradition

The word "mint" doubles for a breath freshening sweet. Altoid being one of the best known brands. But it wasn't originally created as a breath freshener. It was created in 1780 to relieve intestinal discomfort. Though we know now that the sugar in these sweets may offset any medicinal benefit from the peppermint essential oil they contain (Grieves, 1992).

It has been used since ancient times as a remedy for the stomach. The Greeks and Romans would bind it to their head during feasts. I wonder if this was not just for fun but because of its medicinal effects as well. The herb can certainly be used for this.

It is said by Scott Cunningham that if you wear the leaves around your head it will protect against headaches. Seems there was quite a lot of binding herbs to the head back in the day (Cunningham, 2006).

Medicinal Uses

Digestion

Whether it's flatulence, bloating, nausea, heartburn or belching, peppermint does it all. I especially associate peppermint with gas. Whether that's gas that causes flatulence or belching doesn't much matter. This gas can make the stomach bloat and cause griping pains. It's a gentle herb for children with Colic for whom griping pain is a big problem. Some say that it should be used when food is fermenting in the stomach and bowels.

The symptom of gas and flatulence accompanies many gastro-intestinal diseases such as; IBS, Crohn's disease and diverticula. Peppermint can be employed in all of these (Wood, 2008).

Muscles + joints

Its ability to relax muscles in the digestion can be expanded to the whole body and used in problems such as cramps, spasm and muscular pain. For instance, muscle tension can cause backache or stiffness alike. It can also lead to tension headaches and menstrual cramps (Wood, 2008).

Immunity

Peppermint is an interesting herb because it is quite contrary. It's hard to not recognise the taste of mint. It is, rather unusually, heating, but this is followed by a cooling effect. This means it is a rare herb which energises but cools as well. Normally, cooling herbs have a tendency to relax or depress a person, whereas hot herbs energise and uplift someone. The cooling effect of peppermint is especially useful when someone has a fever. Paradoxically, it's specifically used when that fever was brought on by a chill. It is a diaphoretic. This means that it helps to promote sweating with the end effect of lowering body temperature. It also warms the lymphatic system which has the end effect of cooling and moistening the body. The lymph is just one part of the immune system, of course. A major organ that is often forgotten about is the spleen, which makes a lot of good bacteria for the gut as well as white blood cells. Peppermint stimulates the spleen and supports the fight against viruses like *herpes* and shingles. It will also bring down the inflammation of infections such as mastitis (Wood, 2008).

Nerves

Peppermint, despite being stimulating, is also mildly sedating. Another one of its paradoxes. This seeming contradiction is actually a signifier of its changeability which is characterised energetically by wind. In traditional Chinese medicine wind would be characterised by changeability and the appearance of contradiction. It can be used for hysteria. This is an old fashioned term we don't use anymore. It was used to describe a kind of manic nervousness. Usually it was women who were afflicted by it, and probably still are! (Wood, 2008)

Safety Considerations

Do not use in the first trimester of pregnancy. Do not use with those who are anxious, neurotic or excitable. Shouldn't be used in hot, dry conditions of the colon.

—— *Mentha viridis* (spearmint) ——

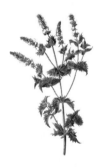

Names: garden mint, mackerel mint, Our Lady's mint, green mint, spire mint, sage of Bethlehem, fish mint, menthe de Notre Dame, erba Santa Maria, lamb mint

Element: Air

Planet: Venus

Magical uses: dream work, connect with male divinity

Key words: fresh, sweet, childhood, comfort

Tissue state: constriction, depression

Qualities: mildly stimulating, warming then cooling

Actions: antispasmodic, carminative, diaphoretic, stimulant

Physical uses: fever, cold, dyspepsia, abdominal cramps, cholera, biliary colic, memory, headache, PCOS, (less powerful than peppermint)

Emotional Uses: cooling a hot head, hysteria, upset children

Parts used: aerial parts

Known constituents: essential oil, flavonoids

Legend and tradition

If you've ever grown mint you'll know it spreads very easily in the UK. But it is actually native to the Mediterranean; it was the Romans who brought mint over to the UK many years ago. It's so common now most would assume it's from here.

The ancients believed mint would prevent the coagulation of milk, thereby preserving it. They also added mint to their baths to improve the smell of the bath and themselves (Grieves, 1992).

Medicinal Uses

Immunity

Spearmint is peppermint's gentler cousin. It stimulates the body but also feels cooling. It'll help bring on a fever so you can sweat off an illness (Grieves, 1992).

Digestion

The essential oils in spearmint help the digestion. It is antispasmodic, which makes it especially good for abdominal cramps and colic (Grieves, 1992).

Reproductive

I also like to use it for painful periods as an essential oil applied to the tummy. But spearmint has a special association with PCOS. It is known to reduce the androgen that is in excess in this condition, leading to symptoms like male pattern hair (Trickey, 2003).

Safety Considerations

None known

—— *Passiflora incarnata* (passionflower) ——

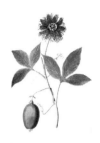

Names: maypop, passion vine, grana-
dilla, maracoc

Element: Water

Planet: Venus

Magical uses: associated with Jupiter and
Uranus (some say Neptune), calms and
brings peace to the house, increases charisma, dream pillows,
love spells, helps promote empathy, to calm a brutal lover,
breaking bad habits fuelled by passions, personal
transformation

Key words: soft, imaginative, divine, spirit, floaty, gentle, deep,
calming, soothing

Tissue state: irritation, constriction

Qualities: cooling, moistening

Actions: anti-inflammatory, hypnotic, vasodilator, antispasmodic, mild sedative, analgesia, hypotensor, tranquilliser,
central nervous system relaxant, strengthens the heart muscle

Physical uses: insomnia due to mental restlessness, nervous
excitability, overactive brain, hyperactive children, hysteria,
alcoholism, twitching of limbs, neuralgia, constrictive headache, tremor (in elderly), benzodiazepine and valium
addiction, rapid heart beat, pain of shingles, anxiety neurosis,
tension, irritability, panic, toothache, period pain, asthma,
palpitations, high blood pressure, muscle cramps

Emotional uses: brings on a dream state, improving clairvoyance and instinct, helps when you're struggling to digest
something, stress and shock, grief, highly strung individuals

Parts used: aerial parts

Known constituents: flavonoids, indole alkaloids, fatty acids, and sterols

Legend and tradition

Passionflower was so named by the Spanish conquistadors, who associated it with Christ. Because of this (and its purple colour) It is associated with divinity and spirituality (Grieves, 1992).

Medicinal uses

Nerves

It is a relaxant and helps to downregulate an overstimulated nervous system. It's perfect for people who overthink or chronically worry, as they can't switch off. These people usually struggle to get to sleep at night because they can't stop thinking about what needs to be done or what's happened in the day. It works on the oblongata that governs sleep, temporary changes of blood pressure and the vagus nerve. I usually get patients who struggle with this type of insomnia to write whatever is on their mind down before trying to sleep (Bartrams, 1995).

Another side effect to an overstimulated nervous system is that the muscles can become spastic. This means they can go in and out of spasm, but they can also get stuck in a chronically tense state as well. If you experience headaches that feel like a weight on your head passionflower is indicated.

Traditionally passionflower was used in more severe cases of spasm such as epilepsy, eclampsia and whooping cough. I wonder about its possible application in the more modern diagnosis; ADHD, as well (Wood, 2008).

Digestion

The connection may not seem obvious but actually the digestive system has as many (if not more) nerves than the brain does. For this reason it's sometimes called the "second brain". It's why, when we're nervous, we sometimes get diarrhoea, and don't want to eat anything. It's also the reason that long-term stress is interlinked with IBS. It's often the missing link that doesn't get made when treating the condition and is perhaps the "secret ingredient" to successfully treating it (Wood, 2008).

It's also good for nervous indigestion, dysentery and was once used for cholera. In fact it's especially nice for diarrhoea in children as it's so gentle but effective. The effects of passionflower seems to be via the vagus nerve, a massive nerve which links the brain to the gut.

Safety Considerations
No known safety considerations

—— *Rhodiola rosea* (rhodiola) ——

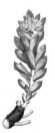

Names: rose root, golden root.

Element: Fire

Planet: Sun

Magical uses: for stamina

Key words: strength, rugged, survival

Tissue state: working on this

Qualities: cooling

Actions: adaptogen, antidepressant, antioxidant, antiviral, immune stimulant, nervine, central nervous system stimulant, antiarrhythmic, neuroprotective

Physical uses: alertness, ADHD, fatigue, memory, depression, immune depletion, altitude sickness, parkinson's, muscle stiffness and spasm, fertility, arrhythmias

Emotional uses: better boundaries, inner strength, confidence

Part used: root

Known constituents: phenols, rosavin, rosin, rosarin, organic acids, terpenoids, phenolic acids, flavonoids, anthraquinones, alkaloids, tyrosol, and salidroside

Legend and tradition

Given to wedding couples for fertility, Vikings used it and recorded it in the first Swedish *Pharmacopaeia* 1775.

Medicinal uses

Nervous

Rhodiola is a herb I remember well for its taste. That drying earthy taste is hard to miss. I used it while studying for my final exams at university. It helps with alertness and memory whilst also calming excited nerves. It makes it useful for ADHD, Parkinson's and muscle spams as a result (Winston & Maimes, 2007).

Circulation

It's said to help with arrhythmias where the heart beats in an irregular fashion (Winston & Maimes, 2007). Again, I'm not so sure this is because it has a direct effect on the cardiovascular system but rather because it calms the excited nerves. This is a good example where knowing the cause of an illness may dictate the herbs that are used and dramatically change the outcome. Herbal medicine usually tries to go as far back in the illnesses journey as it can, while we are used to using drugs that often only go back one or two steps on the symptom. Often people are confused when I tell them that the herb I should suggest depends on the cause, it probably seems like I'm dodging the question. But a single symptom could be treated in a myriad of ways, depending on the cause, when it comes to herbal medicine.

Reproductive

Supporting the nerves and adrenals helps minimise the effect of stress on the body. If you were taking on board earlier chapters you'll already know why. The effects of stress don't end at the adrenals, they affect everything in the body. One area we often take for granted, though, is our fertility. It's really important to minimize stress when trying for babies. This applies to men and women. All the adaptogens can be vital in this battle against modern life. Stress vs. relaxation. Infertility vs. fertility (Winston & Maimes, 2007).

Safety Considerations

I don't recommend using this herb for bipolar, mania, or paranoia. It can cause insomnia in some.

— *Rosa centifolia, damascena and gallica* (rose) —

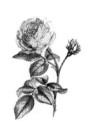

Names: Rose

Element: Water

Planet: Venus

Magical uses: love, psychic powers, healing, divination, luck, protection

Key words: beauty, passion, sweet, love, soft, strong

Tissue state: excitation and relaxation

Qualities: astringent, cooling and aromatic

Actions: mild sedative, mild local anaesthetic, antiinflammatory, laxative, liver protector, antidepressant, aphrodisiac, cardioprotective, cooling skin astringent, increases bile flow, antiviral, menstrual regulator, relaxant, nervine, diuretic, spasmolytic, antiseptic, antiparasitic, digestive, hypolipidemic, and aperient

Physical uses: anaemia, profound anxiety, grief, insomnia, irritability, sore throat, irritated cough, tuberculosis, venous congestion, clotting, poor circulation, thrombosis, angina, diarrhoea, frequent urination, kidney stones, promotes bile, cleanse gallbladder, vaginitis, leucorrhoea, painful periods, heavy periods, irregular periods, infertility, libido, arthritis, fatigue, virus

Emotional uses: love, opens heart chakra, traumatic births, grief, antidepressant, combats apathy, nourishes the heart, lifts the spirit, evokes sexual bliss

Parts used: petals, flower heads

Known constituents: tannins, flavonoids, carotene, essential oils, anthocyanidins, vitamins C, B, E, K, fatty oils, nicotinamide

Legend and tradition

Roses grow all over the world. There are records of rose being used in Persia as early as 500 BC and fossilised roses have been found which are over 35 million years old, while the oldest rose living today has been alive since 815 AD! To have a flower essence of that Rose would surely heal all the ills of the world (Grieves, 1992).

The Romans would suspend a bunch of roses above a table to show that whatever was said beneath was in confidence. That's why the beautiful botanical plaster designs around the central light fixtures in ceilings are called "the rose". This is also why the term, *sub rosa*, means "in secret".

Sufi's in Islam also use it as a symbol for divine love. The Greeks used it as a strong representative of Aphrodite and then the Romans used it for Venus.

Medicinal uses

Traditionally the petals, sepals, hips, leaves, stalks, roots, root bark and thorns were all used as medicine. But now, we only use the hips (fruit) of the *Rosa canina* and the petals of the *Rosa centifolia* and *damascena*.

Cardiovascular

Rose helps to support the cardiovascular system by strengthening blood vessels and reducing bad cholesterol. It helps when some-one bruises too easily, gets blood clots, or has poor circulation from congestion in the arteries. This in turn helps with more severe problems, such as angina. It has even been used to improve blood quality in cases of anaemia, though it is not clear to me by what mechanism this occurs (Wood, 2008).

Digestion

The rose can be used to support digestion as well. Its tannins help to heal the gut wall and tone the gut where it has become too "floppy" to truly absorb food correctly. In some cases of diarrhoea, where the intestines are actually moving very quickly but not absorbing the food, rose will help to calm this down. Traditionally this would be seen as an excited tissue state and rose is helpful in calming it (Wood, 2008).

Immunity

Rose helps to relieve the heat of this excitation and aids people who have rheumatism and arthritis. The Native Americans also used it for influenza, stomach upsets and fevers. Which makes me wonder if rose has some antiviral properties or is good at supporting the immune system in a less direct way. Its effect may be found through its ability to support the stress response, for instance (Wood, 2008).

Nerves

Rose could help support someone in those situations but it is best with the side effects of long-term excitation such as fatigue, asthenia, and insomnia. It is also good for but fatigue, convalescence, asthenia, anaemia, children wetting the bed, profound anxiety, insomnia, and irritability (Wood, 2008).

Lungs

I had never thought of rose being associated with the lungs until researching this monograph. The tea can be used for tuberculosis (though we wouldn't do that now), sore throats (thanks to the tanins) and back in 1919 George Slack used it for bleeding from the lungs (again we would go to hospital for that now) (Wood, 2008).

Reproductive

Rose has a strong association with the feminine, including the hormonal cycle. It is wonderful for balancing the menstrual cycle. It helps to relieve premenstrual tension, melts frigidity and eases menopausal symptoms. It is especially well known for helping to cool menopausal hot flushes. When used externally it helps inflammation and itching such as vaginal itching, especially during the menopause. It is also useful when itching is due to infection such as yeast overgrowth. Often cases of cystitis accompany thrush imbalances and rose is useful for both. When there is an unusual discharge from the vagina with no known cause it is called leucorrhea, and this is aided by rose. It also helps with irregular periods, heavy periods and infertility (Trickey, 2003).

Safety Considerations

No known safety considerations

—— *Rosmarianus officinalis* (rosemary) ——

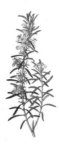

Names: polar plant, compass-weed, compass plant, *Rosmarianus coronarium*

Element: Fire

Planet: Sun

Magical uses: protection against nightmares, protection against evil, love, lust, mental powers, unification and sleep

Key words: hot, pungent, spikey, clear, poke, evergreen, strong

Tissue state: atrophy and depression

Qualities: hot and dry

Actions: antibacterial, antidepressant, antispasmodic, antiseptic, circulatory tonic, diffusive stimulant, diuretic, sedative, mild substitute for Benzodiazepine drugs

Physical uses: arteriosclerosis, migraines, hypertension, palpitations, headache from gastric upset, occipital tension, psychogenic depression, cardiac debility, giddiness, hyperactivity, tremor of limbs, cholecystitis, yellow complexion, slow digestion, strengthen blood vessels, chronic fatigue syndrome, low energy, strengthens intestines, swellings, gout, congestive heart disease, cardiac oedema, bruises, stiffness, soreness, arthritis, strains, epilepsy, apoplexies, palsies, hair loss, sinusitis, bronchitis, dry heaving, bloating, vomiting, high cholesterol, obesity, amenorrhoea, leucorrhea, prevents miscarriage, post-partum depression, hot flashes, gastric reflux

Emotional uses: compass weed helps you find yourself again, find your path, self-hood, insecurity, gives clarity, warmth and inner peace

Parts used: leaves and flowers

Known constituents: flavonoids, proanthocyanidins, tannins, terpenoid bitters, phenols, acids, volatile oils, resin, camphor

Legend and tradition

Rosemary is the herb of remembrance. Coming from the Mediterranean, it was prized by Arabic physicians. But has been native in the UK for a long time now. During the times of the plague it was put in the hands of the dead before they were buried. Some say years after a rosemary bush would have grown over the coffin. Perhaps this is something we can look for the next time we walk through a cemetery. It symbolised the immortality of the soul and would have comforted the mourners. It may have had a more practical use at funerals too, as it was said to protect against the plague and may have helped protect the living from whatever disease the dead person had died from (Grieves, 1992).

In Greece, students would entwine rosemary in their hair to help them remember what they were learning. Even today people burn rosemary essential oil to help with studying and taking exams. I remember I did at school, following my mum's advice.

Medicinal Uses

Rosemary will make you burn through what energy you have faster. Matthew Wood thinks of rosemary as oxygenating the body, thereby increasing its burning processes. It actually increases metabolism and helps with fat absorption. It aids those with high cholesterol too.

Nerves

But the stimulating effects of rosemary are not akin to that of, say, coffee. While coffee can make us feel wired and has a nasty come-down for some, rosemary does not. It actually stimulates the parasympathetic nervous system, which is responsible for the rest and relax response, while also relaxing the sympathetic nervous system which is responsible for our flight and fight response. A sensible and complementary set of actions. But, like coffee, it can be used to help you wake in the morning. In fact, it might stop you from sleeping if you have it close to your bed time (Brooke, 1992).

Cardiovascular

Rosemary helps remove congealed blood, as in the case of bruises. It also helps to open the capillaries, which can help with tension headaches and migraines. It strengthens the blood vessels, which helps in cases of arteriosclerosis as well as hypertension. But it is best to see a herbalist before using rosemary in cases of those with hypertension, as it can make it worse for people with a sanguine constitution. Constitutions are hard to assess, even by the experienced herbalist (Brooke, 1992).

Juliette de Bairacli Levy describes rosemary as the perfect herb for congestive heart failure. She puts this down to three actions which it has: it is cleansing, it is a nervine and it is toning. She recommends it as a tea with honey for optimum effect.

Musculoskeletal

One of the more marked effects of rosemary, especially in a tea, is how drying it is on the tongue. This drying effect is indicative that it would not be suitable in conditions which are already hot, such as dry eczemas. However, in what may seem a contradiction, it is useful for arthritis. Arthritis is an inflammatory condition of the joints. But there are two types: osteoarthritis and rheumatoid arthritis. It's rarely helpful in the case of rheumatoid arthritis where the body is attacking itself via. a heightened immune system. It is far more useful for cases of osteoarthritis where there is wear and tear. Specifically, keep an ear out for people whose symptoms are worsened by cold and damp conditions (Wood, 2008).

Digestion and elimination

I mentioned before that rosemary helps with the absorption of fats. It has other actions on the digestive system too. It also aids in dry heaving and vomiting. It supports the spleen, liver and kidney so it would aid a detoxing action on the body (Wood, 2008).

Reproduction

Another situation in which rosemary's drying capacity is useful is in the case of leucorrhea (Brooke, 1992). This is a white or yellowish discharge from the vagina. It has many causes but the most common is high oestrogen. It also helps with the quality and flow of blood in the womb. Rosemary can help initiate the flow of blood for those who have gone a long time without periods. But, it also has been used traditionally to prevent miscarriage. I do wonder what dosage they were using for this action as I would be concerned about the high volatile oil content of the plant during pregnancy, as it may have an abortifacient action. Penelope Ody warns against its use in pregnancy at medicinal doses but feels normal culinary use is perfectly safe. Its stimulating effects have also been used traditionally to lift the mood for women if they suffer postpartum depression. But again, I would prefer to use things like oat tops and nettle to do this because of the drying effects that rosemary has.

Safety Considerations

Because of the heating action of rosemary it's important to only use it in the right sort of people. Although it can be used to treat hypertension it may also make it worse for those who are of the full-blooded sanguine nature. It can also be too stimulating for people who are very nervous. Both of these types of people probably need something more gentle first. Whenever I use rosemary it probably makes up no more than five percent of a prescription, it is so powerful. Rosemary is safe in culinary doses during pregnancy, but not as a tincture or as medicinal infusions.

—— *Rubus ideaus* (raspberry leaf) ——

Names: raspbis, hindberry, bramble of Mount Ida, hindbeer

Element: Water

Planet: Venus

Magical uses: protection, love. Hang branches over the door for protection and to stop the spirit of the deceased from returning to the house

Key words: sweet, strength, power, stamina, prickle, dry

Tissue state: relaxation, excitation, atrophy

Qualities: astringent

Actions: astringent tonic, antispasmodic, parturient, galactagogue, relaxant, partus preparatus, febrifuge

Physical uses: irregular menstruation, painful periods, preparation for birth, increase breast milk supply, after-birth pains, prostate health, low libido in men, male sterility, baldness, mouth ulcers, sore throat, strep throat, tonsilitis, vaginal discharge, nausea during pregnancy, diarrhoea, phlegm in upper respiratory tract, flu with gut involvement, gastrointestinal haemorrhage, diverticular disease, dysentry, colic, chronic Constipation, nervousness, cataract, canker sores, teething, post nasal drip, scars, fever

Emotional uses: helps you feel childish again, strengthens parent/child bonds, improves clairvoyance and activates root chakra.

Parts used: leaves

Known constituents: fragrine, volatile oils, tannin, minerals including potassium, ferric acid (a type of iron), calcium, magnesium and zinc as well as vitamins including vits A, B, C & E.

Legend and tradition

It is thought that the name, *ideaus*, comes from the place name where it was supposedly originally found; Mount Ida. This was in Ancient Greece and is now Turkey. The other theory about the name *idaeus* comes from Greek mythology. According to the myth, the berries were white until a nymph, Ida pricked her finger while picking them. From then on the fruits were coloured red with her blood. It has even been found by archaeologists in old Roman and Greek settlements, where it was likely they used it as much for medicine as they did for food. Before its modern name, raspberry, it was sometimes called hindberry (Grieves, 1992).

Medicinal uses

Although raspberry is famed for its use in pregnancy, as a way to prepare the womb for labour, this is quite a modern use. For hundreds of years before that it was used primarily for its astringent properties (Trickey, 2003).

Digestion

The leaves help to dry diarrhoea and I once used blackberry (the more astringent sister plant) to help a patient experiencing blood in the stools. This is a symptom they should have seen their doctor about urgently, but the patient refused. I was very pleased the blackberry leaf helped. The fruit used to be eaten in large quantities to help with constipation, increase sweating and ease rheumatism and indigestion (Grieves, 1992).

Reproduction

In modern times it is best known, and most widely used, for its benefits during labour. Two famous British herbalists, Thomson and Coffin, are said to record the earliest use of the herb as preparation for birth. Rather than using it before the birth they used it during labour itself, but I recommend women drink 1–3 cups in the last trimester to tone the muscles gradually. It was once thought that it achieved this action by being mainly contractive to muscle tissue. However, it has been tested and discovered to be a relaxant to the uterine muscles. Therefore, it has been hypothesised that it helps by orchestrating the contraction of the muscles in unity. A lack of coordination in the muscles is thought to lie behind why some women "fail to progress" during labour (Trickey, 2003).

Interestingly this action on the muscles of the uterus during pregnancy does not seem to occur outside of pregnancy. This was quite confounding when discovered as raspberry leaf can be used to relieve heavy and painful periods. Ruth Trickey (2003) argues that it may be helpful in heavy periods because of its iron, vitamins and other mineral content.

Its toning effects makes it useful not only during pregnancy but also afterwards for the healing process while the body realigns.

Safety Considerations
Avoid during the first trimester of pregnancy

—— *Sambucus nigra* (elder) ——

Names: devil's eye, lady elder, Frau Holle, tree of doom, old lady, Lady Ellhorn, whistle tree, pipe tree, black elder, bore tree, bour tree, hylder, hylantree, eldrum, ellhorn, *hollunder* (German), *sureau* (French), the elder mother, the queen of herbs, old lady, Old Sal

Element: Air

Planet: Venus

Magical uses: wands, head dress at Beltane, to see spirits, Holda, Hecate, healing, Protection, exorcism, prosperity, wish manifestation

Key words: lifting, mystic, dark, deep, rich, light, fluffy

Tissue state: used for irritation and constriction. Dry flowers; depression. Berries; atrophy

Qualities: moist and cool. Sedative and stimulant

Actions: diaphoretic, anti-inflammatory, antirheumatic, astringent, antiviral, antibacterial, vulnerary, laxative (berries and bark), anticatarrhal, hydragogue (inner bark), cathartic (inner bark), emollient (flowers), diuretic (flowers), expectorant (flowers), sudorific (flowers), febrifuge (flowers), anodyne (flowers)

Physical uses: **Berries** and **flowers**: coughs, colds, congestion, cllergies, crthritis, *candidiasis*, earache, flu, sinusitis, tonsillitis, night sweats, chilblains, kidney stones, weepy eczema, weepy ulcers, colic, diarrhoea, rheumatism, syphilis, headaches, sciatica. **leaves**: insect repellant when bruised, ointment for bruises, sprains, chilblains, purgative, diuretic, diaphoretic; **bar**k: strong purgative, ointment relieves asthma and croup; **flowers**: lightens freckles, bronchitis, pulmonary affections, fever management, blood purifier, oedema, gout

Emotional uses: the flower lifts the spirits, mild antidepressant, grief, nightmares, childhood night terrors

Parts used: berries and flowers internally. Leaves externally only

Known constituents: flavonoids, phenolic acid, triterpenes, sterols, volatile oils, mucilage, tannins; **Berries**: anthocyanins, vitamins A and C. **leaves**: Cyanogenic glycosides

Legend and tradition

The Danish sometimes refer to the tree as *Hylde Moer* meaning "Elder Mother", referring to the spirit of a witch that is said to live within the tree. To cut into an Elder was to invoke the witch's wrath upon you. It is said in Britain that a witch-tree once turned an invading Danish king into stone, creating the Rollright Stones in Oxfordshire.

Gypsies would carefully avoid it when kindling a fire but it's name is thought to derive from i's potential use in doing just that, *Æld* being Anglo-Saxon for fire (Grieves, 1992).

Medicinal Uses

The flower

The flowers of the elder are such a sight to behold. From a distance they look like fluffy clouds of cream on the tree. Believed to mark the beginning of summer in the UK, the berries mark the end. The flowers are usually at their best around midsummer and should be picked while in full bloom.

Immunity

The most common use for elderflower is probably during a cold or flu. It's excellent for many of the symptoms associated with these. It can be used to reduce a fever by promoting a sweat (sudorific). You can't have too much really but it's important to always keep a careful watch on someone with a fever in case it goes up into dangerous territory.

The elderflower can be used to break down mucous in the lungs so you can get rid of it when you cough (Brooke, 1992). It'll also break down mucous if you find yourself feeling blocked up in the nose too. The best way to deal with this is to use it as an inhalation.

Musculoskeletal

Its cooling effect is also good in cases of rheumatism and gout. These are both very painful conditions affecting the joints. The painful sensation is caused by inflammation. It can also be used for pain caused by sciatica.

The berry

The properties of the berry are very similar to the flower but they're also thought to be a tonic and blood building. This means they help add to the quality of blood. Especially in anemia.

There's a lot of scare mongering around elder at the moment. I'm not sure where it came from. But many are being told that it is poisonous. Some of it *is* poisonous if you have *enough* of it. Best thing to do is to avoid consuming any green parts. Having said that, I have a friend that once juiced about a kilo of fresh berries and consumed it in one go. This made her vomit. A highly prized healing response back in the day! An unpleasant side effect now. Nevertheless, she wasn't poisoned (Brooke, 1992).

Vomiting would have been used to lessen certain humours in the days before doctors. In fact, elder has all the detoxing actions rolled into one plant so it could have been used for any humour. It was thought to have all the healing properties needed for any ailment and planted in gardens across the UK for this reason. It is an emetic (makes you vomit), diaphoretic (makes you sweat), laxative, diuretic (makes you wee), expectorant (makes you cough up phlegm) and emmenagogue (starts a period).

The leaf

Skin

I know the leaf best for its anti-inflammatory properties externally on the skin for things like bites and stings. I usually infuse it in a base oil and make a balm. The leaves are diuretic, expectorant and purgative. These uses would have been employed in the past but we're not as risk averse as our ancestors were (Bartrams, 1995).

Safety Considerations

Don't consume any green part of the plant: leaves, bark, stem

—— *Scutellaria lateriflora* (skullcap) ——

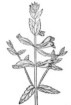

Names: quaker bonnet, mad-dog skullcap, madweed

Element: Earth

Planet: Saturn

Magical uses: bind oaths, consecrate vows

Key words: calm, head space

Tissue state: constrictive, atrophy, excitation

Qualities: relaxing, bitter

Actions: antispasmodic, anticonvulsive, nervine, vasodilator, sedative

Physical uses: headache, migraine, PMS, insomnia, nervous stress or shock

Emotional uses: overwhelmed, everything on top of you, pressure from inside or outside

Parts used: aerial parts

Known constituents: flavonoid glycosides, scutellarin, tannins, iridoids

Legend and tradition

The name skullcap comes from the latin *scutella*, which describes the appearance of the lid of the calyx. Its names "mad-dog skullcap" and "madweed" come from the belief that it is a cure for hydrophobia (Grieves, 1992).

Medicinal uses

Nervous

I've always thought of skullcap as being associated with the head.

Why not, with a name like that? But through my research for this book, it has come to light that this is a bastardisation of the name's origins. Having said that, it certainly helps you remember what it does! Aiding with headaches, migraines and insomnia, calming the nervous system and allowing healing to occur (Wood, 2008).

Reproductive

This is another herb I'd use for PMS. It helps to calm and soothe the nervous system that feels ragged and raw during the premenstrual phase.

Safety Considerations

No known safety considerations

—— *Taraxacum officinale* (dandelion) ——

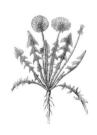

Names: priests crown, swine's snout, dent de lion, *dens leonis* (a lions tooth), *Leontodon* (greek), piss-a-bed, fortune teller, cankerwort, wet-weed, time teller, wishes

Element: Air

Planet: Jupiter

Magical uses: divination, calling spirits, making wishes, contacting Hecate, enhances psychic abilities, brings favourable winds, association with Samhain and Beltane, balances the self, invokes sylphs and air spirits

Key words: detox, ground, Hecate, Samhain, Beltane, spring, autumn, darkness

Tissue state: used for stagnation, cold and dry

Actions: diuretic, hepatic, cholagogue, galactagogue, pancreatic regulator, urinary antiseptic, anti-eczema, detoxifying, antirheumatic, laxative, tonic, bitter

Physical uses: **root**: romotes elimination of plasma cholesterol, liver tonic, inflammation of liver and gallbladder, gallstones, mild jaundice, hangovers, constipation, indigestion, lack of appetite, hypoglycaemia, anorexia nervosa, congestive heart failure, diabetes, anaemia, hepatits, liver heat, skin problems such as acne, eczema, boils, age spots, abscesses, and *herpes*; **leaf**: kidney tonic, lower blood pressure and replenish potassium levels, fluid retention, sweating in between the bum cheeks, muscular rheumatism, warts, promotes weight loss during dieting, oedema

Emotional uses: grounding, releasing anger, releasing pent-up emotions, reducing liver-heat, reducing depression and self-hate, increasing self-care, better sense of self.

Parts used: root and leaf medicinally. The flowers are edible. The juice from the stem can be used topically, not internally

Known constituents: Sesquiterpene lactones, triterpenes, vitamins A, B, C and D, phytosterols, flavanoids, polysaccharides; **leaf only:** carotenoids, coumarins, minerals, especially potassium; **root only:** taraxcoside, phenolic acids, minerals such as potassium and calcium

Legend and tradition

The name dandelion, which most of us know it by, comes from *dent-de-lion*, which is French for "lions tooth". This is a reference to the sharp jagged edge of the leaf. Not, as I once thought, the yellow petals, which also look like a lion's mane. It was also called *piss en lit* by the French, meaning "piss-the-bed". This was in reference to its diuretic properties. In fact, some adults and children alike will still remember being told they would pee the bed at night if they touched a dandelion. Although it does help you pass urine it would be rather remarkable an effect for it to occur simply by touching it! (Grieves, 1992)

Medicinal uses

The root

Digestion and elimination

The root is bitter, more so than the leaves. This bitterness gives it some of its wonderful health benefits. Bitter tastes help to stimulate the digestive system by making the pancreas produce more bile. This helps us digest our food more effectively. It also helps us excrete waste products more efficiently (Bartrams, 1995).

However, its ability to speed up the transit time of the liver means that even medications from the doctor, if we are taking them, will be processed faster. For this reason you could say that the drugs will have less of an effect. It's important for those on medication to seriously reconsider using dandelion because of this (Wood, 2008).

As a herb of Jupiter, dandelion root can be used to help with any disease of the liver. It's traditionally used for things such as mild jaundice, gallstones and cirrhosis of the liver (Brooke, 1992).

Because the root is so good at helping the liver function it can help with conditions which come about through an over-burdened liver. For example, skin conditions such as eczema and psoriasis can be aided by helping the liver.

Thanks to the roots effects on the liver and bile production it also helps those who suffer with constipation. Firstly by increasing the breakdown of food products. Secondly, by improving the movement in the intestines.

Cardiovascular

Although it's not usually thought of as supportive to the cardiovascular system, it does help with swollen hands and feet which can be a symptom of congestive heart failure. It also helps support the cardiovascular system by clearing bad cholesterol (Wood, 2008).

Endocrine

Dandelion root is also great for balancing blood sugar levels. This may make it a great addition to any blend for balancing hormones in women who are oestrogen dominant (e.g. endometriosis) as well as for those suffering with type 2 diabetes. Women will also find it useful if they suffer with symptoms, such as spots that occur as part of their hormone cycle or migraines associated with their cycle (Brooke, 1992).

The leaf

Urinary

While the root is associated with the liver, the leaf is associated with the kidneys. As a remedy for the kidney it is great for lowering high blood pressure. This is because the volume of blood we produce is monitored by the kidneys. When we support the kidney we support the heart in turn. What's wonderful about dandelion is that, while prescribed diuretics used to deplete potassium levels, dandelion does not. However, having said that, in recent times diuretic drugs have been corrected so this depletion is no longer the case (Grieves, 1992).

Not only does the leaf affect the kidneys, it also affects the bladder. As we have already mentioned it is known as a diuretic for children. Its ability to improve the filtration rate of the kidneys means the bladder also excretes urine more often. This is extremely useful in cases of cystitis, urethritis and kidney stones (Grieves, 1992).

Cardiovascular

Traditionally, dandelion is seen as a blood cleanser. This action is partially through its action on the liver but also through its action on the kidneys that, of course, filter the blood for waste products that need to be excreted. As a result it can help with conditions such as arthritis, rheumatism and gout (Wood, 2008).

Lungs

Dandelion is less known for its effect on the lungs but Elizabeth

Brooke and Matthew Wood mention it as being useful for the lungs, for chronic coughs, asthma and bronchitis, as it strengthens the lung tissues (Brooke, 1992).

Safety considerations

Do not give to those on medication for blood pressure, especially if it is low. Could be dangerous to those with a history of family allergy. Contact dermatitis is sometimes seen in response to the juice in the stem.

Do not give while the bile duct is blocked or before gall stone sizes have been identified. You can block the gall bladder by using bitters to clear stones if they're too big.

Do not use while on medication which is treating a chronic illness or which needs to be taken daily such as the contraceptive pill.

—— *Thymus vulgaris* (thyme) ——

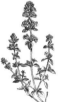

Names: common thyme

Element: Air

Planet: Venus

Magical uses: banish fear, courage, call upon fairy folk, light heartedness when working hard to achieve your dreams

Key words: uplift, energize, rising

Tissue state: depressed, constriction, atrophy and stagnation

Qualities: hot, dry, stimulating

Actions: antiseptic, antibacterial, antioxidant, antifungal, antitussive, antispasmodic, axpectorant, aiaphoretic, anthelmintic, carminative, diuretic, mild sedative, anti-candida, antiviral

Physical uses: respiratory infections, sinusitis, strep throat, gingivitis, laryngitis, painful or late periods, mastitis, leucorrhea, nightmare, headache, hangover, parasites, gout, rheumatism

Emotional uses: courage, strength to hold on, life traumas

Parts used: leaves

Known constituents: tannins, gums, flavonoids, volatile oils, caffeic acid

Caution: pregnancy

Legend and tradition

Embroidered on handerkerchief, given to knights for protection, symbol of republicanism. (Grieves, 1992)

Medicinal uses

Immunity

Thyme is one of the strongest antivirals I use. It gets chucked at most things; sinusitis, strep throat, gingivitis, laryngitis, you name it. It's best when applied to illness affecting the upper respiratory system but I had a colleague who used it against MRSA and found it effective (Brooke, 1992).

Natural antivirals often make mincemeat of the super-bugs we've become so afraid of. Some think it's because the herbs have so many constituents in them it's hard for the bacteria to resist, others think it's simply because they haven't been overprescribed. I hope more research is done in this area, and fast!

Reproductive

The moving ability of the volatile oils in thyme make it great for stimulating a late period to begin. But also, it should be avoided during pregnancy for this reason. Its antiviral properties make it useful for mastitis and it is helpful for candida and leucorrhea where there is a bacterial overgrowth of some sort. Often with bacterial overgrowths you need to experiment for a while to get the exact right herb that helps. But if the problem is fairly new you may find that thyme is useful as the body won't be accustomed to it yet (Wood, 2008).

Nervous

Thyme is quite stimulating, helping with debility and fatigue. I would avoid using it in chronic fatigue though, where the person needs nourishing before stimulating. You can't pour from an empty cup. For the same reason these people should avoid stimulants like sugar and caffeine (Grieves, 1992).

Musculoskeletal

Can be used in gout and rheumatism

Safety Considerations

Do not use during pregnancy or lactation

—— *Tilia cordata* (lime blossom) ——

Names: linden flowers, linn flowers, common lime

Element: Air

Planet: Jupiter and Venus

Magical uses: associated with the planet Jupiter, the element of air and the astrological symbol Venus. Used magically to strengthen protection magic. It will help to enhance your luck, especially in love and makes a great addition to any spell cast for sleep problems

Key words: cooling, calming, soothing, comforting, strong, gentle, heart, tummy

Tissue state: atrophy and irritation

Qualities: cooling and moistening

Actions: antispasmodic, diaphoretic, diuretic, sedative, hypotensive, anticoagulant, anxiolytic & immune enhancer

Physical uses: stress, fever, indigestion, nervousness, hyperactivity, insomnia, anxiety, panic, nervous vomiting, colic, diarrhoea, cramp, arteriosclerosis, hypertension, oedema, pelvic inflammatory disease, uterine pain, vulvodynia, fever, skin irritation, spasm, sores, herpes, shingles, cold sores, migraine and headaches or pain, acute illness

Emotional uses: comforting, nervousness, warms a frozen heart

Parts used: flowers

Known constituents: flavonoids, tannins, amino acids, mucilaginous, polysaccharides, sterols, steroidal saponins, phenolic acids and volatile oils

Legend and tradition

Hildegard von Bingen used a talisman of lime to ward off the plague. The talisman was made with a green stone covering lime flowers that were wrapped in a spider's web (Grieves, 1992).

Medicinal uses

Nerves

Lime flowers are best known for their calming effect but more traditionally it was used as a remedy for convulsions and epilepsy, even in children. I wouldn't recommend that you try to use lime blossom for this use now though, as the drugs available may be more reliable. In terms of energetics epilepsy and convulsions often arise from an excited and constricted tissue state; lime blossom is a relaxant and therefore opposes that (Wood, 2008).

Immunity

As a relaxant to the excited tissue state, lime blossom also helps in cases of hyperactivity, ADD and ADHD. Excitation of the tissue can be thought of like boiling water. When water gets heated the molecules start to move about and bump into each other. The heat and the movement go hand in hand. When something moves a lot it causes heat as well. When the body becomes hot and irritated with excitation it can produce a fever. Despite being hot it is also leads the body into a natural cooling mechanism as the body will sweat to bring the temperature back down. If a fever is becoming uncomfortable you can use something called antipyretics (antifire) in herbal medicine. Lime will help to break a fever in and calm the shivers of influenza as well. It also helps to clear coughs which accompany colds especially when caused by mucous in the lungs (Brooke, 1992).

Nerves

Sometimes constriction and excitation can lead to headaches and migraine. Lime is helpful in this situation, especially when stress is a contributing factor. If stress leads to nervousness, insomnia, restlessness, panic attacks, anxiety or palpitations lime is a great idea (Brooke, 1992).

Cardiovascular

A lot of these symptoms involve the cardiovascular system and it can be used to help more serious problems such as high blood pressure (hypertension) (Bartrams, 1995). I used it with a patient who had a heart defect along with hawthorn, dandelion root and motherwort to help manage their irregular heartbeat till they could have surgery. In fact, we found that their cholesterol levels dropped as well.

Digestion

It's becoming apparent, as we research the digestive system more, that there is a link in the nervous system between the brain and the gut. Most of us will have experienced the effects of stress on our tummies. Not only does lime help with stress is also helps with wind, colic, diarrhoea, indigestion and nervous vomiting (Wood, 2008).

Reproductive

Another way that constriction can express itself is through cramps. When women experience bad cramps with their period lime may be helpful. It will help to lower inflammation in the pelvis (including pelvic inflammatory disease), uterus, and genitalia as a whole, which is why it's used for vulvodynia (Trickey, 2003).

Obviously, cramps can be quite painful. I've used lime blossom in teas many times to help reduce pain. Pain is often caused by inflammation which it combats and is worsened by feeling anxiety around the pain. In fact, it's thought that there is primary and secondary pain. Primary pain being the pain caused by the actual problem. While secondary is the pain which is added to that because of the worry about what the pain means or the apprehension that the pain may get worse. Essentially we make our pain levels go up by worrying about it. Not only have I used it for pain post-surgery but it can also be used in chronic pain like neuralgia.

Skin

Lastly, lime flowers are also helpful for the skin, and this is another area where it cools inflammation. It is helpful in cases of burning eruptions, sores, shingles, *herpes* and even psoriasis. Maybe next time you get some sort of irritated skin rash you can reach for lime leaves instead of aloe vera gel! (Brooke, 1992)

Safety Considerations
None known

—— *Urtica dioica* (nettle) ——

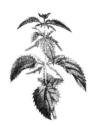

Names: stinging nettle, common nettle, *grosse brennessel* (German), *grande ortie* (French), *ortega* (Spanish), *grande optic* (Italian)

Element: Fire

Planet: Mars

Magical uses: cleansing athames, dye for Ostara eggs (Easter eggs), protection, healing, lust, exorcism, banishing curses. Blend with yarrow to rid yourself of fear

Key words: sting, hot, ouch! strength, boundaries, oomph, power

Tissue state: use for depression, stagnation and atrophy

Qualities: hot and dry

Actions: tonic, haemostatic, lactagogue / galactagogue, diuretic, astringent, anti-allergic, anti-inflammatory tonic to blood, hypoglycaemic, antiseptic, expectorant, vasodilator, hypotensive, antirheumatic, anti-haemorrhagic

Physical uses: tonic, allergies, arthritis, gout, phlegm, lung irritations, urticaria, cleansing, stops heavy menstrual bleeding, promotes breast milk, iron deficiency anaemia, insulin resistant diabetes, paralysis, impotence, atrophy, hypothyroidism, excessive menstruation, loss of hair, bad memory, low blood pressure, bronchitis, asthma, hayfever, cystitis, urethritis, prostatitis, enlarged prostate, burns, hives, blood in stool, itching

Emotional uses: raise the fire in you, improved personal boundaries, gives passion

Parts used: leaves, roots and seeds

Known constituents: tannins, iron, vitamins A, B, C and K, quercetin, histamine, choline, acetylcholine, serotonin

Legend and tradition

Nettle is a fiery plant, as evidenced by its sting. When the Romans came to Britain for the first time it was used to keep themselves warm by stuffing their trousers with it. Sounds like agony, but Britain was much colder then. It just goes to show how desperate they were to stay warm. It was also used to whip the joints following saunas to keep the joints mobile. It's still used to this day to keep away rheumatism. Its Latin name *Urtica* comes from *Uro* meaning "I burn" and its common name nettle comes from the Old English word *noedle* meaning "needle" (Grieves, 1992).

Medicinal uses
The leaf

Nettle is a natural superfood, rich in vitamins A, B, C, D and K. Therefore, I think of it as a superfood. It is traditional to pick the leaf in spring time as a tonic, but it can be picked all year round provided you keep pruning back older growth to promote new young leaves. This is important because the older leaves (the ones still there while it flowers and seeds) are not only more vicious with their stings and more woody in texture but also contain something called a cystolith. This is a tiny molecule which you absorb when you eat the nettle and can contribute to rheumatism, arthritis, gall stones and kidney stones. The irony is that the younger leaf is known to *treat* these conditions (Brooke, 1992).

I feel that the effects of the cystoliths may be slow to build and therefore I only actively avoid the mature plant in people who have a genetic predisposition for any of the illnesses it can contribute to or are currently suffering with one.

Cardiovascular

The superfood properties of nettle makes it useful in treating anemia. This is a state of low iron in the blood. It can be caused by having lost blood but can also contribute to losing more blood. For example, if a woman has a heavy period she will lose blood and her iron levels will reduce. As a result of this she is more likely to bleed heavily the next time too, creating a self-perpetuating cycle. Nettle helps replace the iron which has been lost, while also reducing the likelihood of bleeding. But this is not just true of the womb but also the stomach, and intestines if they are bleeding. Though I should add that if you are vomiting or defecating blood, especially if it's bright red, you should seek emergency help immediately. I give it to women throughout their pregnancies as it is common to become anaemic during pregnancy. Women also bleed after having given birth, so more blood is lost. It also helps prevent haemorrhage during childbirth (Wood, 2008).

Nettle is a lovely herb for women after giving birth, since it helps to increase breast milk supply. My theory is that it does this by ensuring the woman is fully nourished, as breast milk is difficult to produce when you are deficient in vitamins and minerals. I'd recommend making 2–3 cups of the tea each day throughout pregnancy and beyond to utilise its nutritional / medicinal benefit.

Immunity

Taken internally as a tea or tincture the nettle leaf is effective against many allergies. I use it to reduce hay fever, eczema and asthma alike. But it is more traditional to use it in a cream for the skin in cases of eczema, itching and rashes. It's also useful in rheumatism, which is a form of inflammation affecting the joints. I see nettle as a herb which reduces a hyperactive immune system but it is always worth combining it with other cooling herbs in cases of chronic inflammation, because it is hot and dry in quality and could aggravate some conditions (Wood, 2008).

Urinary

The leaf has an affinity for the kidney and bladder and has a diuretic effect (Grieves, 1992). This means it will increase the efficiency with which you produce urine. This is really helpful in reducing hypertension, cystitis, gall stones, kidney disease and hyperglycaemia. It's a very gentle but effective herb and I've yet to find a person that doesn't suit it.

The root
Reproduction
Close by to the kidney and bladder is the prostate gland. This can become enlarged and enflamed in men. In fact, as many as forty percent of men will get it at some point after they reach forty years old. The leaf is helpful but the root even more so. A decoction is best suited for roots. Take it 1–2 times a day (1 tsp per cup) or 5ml a day of tincture will suffice (Brooke, 1992).

The seed
Endocrine
This is a rarely used part of the plant. Though it is coming to be used more by modern herbalists due to its apparent adaptogenic nature. This means that it seems to help people adapt to stress.

Safety considerations
Possible allergy to the sting. Possible allergy to the urticacaea.

—— *Withania somnifera* (ashwagandha) ——

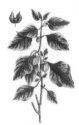

Names: winter cherry, asgandh

Element: Fire / Earth

Planet: Mars

Magical uses: love and romance

Key words: strength, vigor, relaxation

Tissue state: atrophy, constriction, excitation

Qualities: warming, relaxing

Actions: adaptogen, anti-inflammatory, antioxidant, immune support, anti-tumor, nervine, antispasmodic, mild astringent, diuretic

Physical uses: malnutrition, gastric ulcers, debility, fatigue, paralysis, calming adaptogen, anaemia, cloudy thinking, anxiety, coughs, asthma, fevers, infertility, oedema

Emotional uses: builds stamina and inner strength, emotional resilience, turns overactive ego into humility, confidence

Parts used: root

Known constituents: steroidal lactones, alkaloids

Legend and tradition

Asgandh in hindi meaning "horse sweat-like odour". Gives stamina of a horse, enhancing vigour (Winston & Maimes, 2007).

Medicinal uses

Nervous

Although I like to favour British herbs that I can get hold of locally or grow myself, ashwagandha is an exception. It is wonderful for helping with the debility and fatigue that I see all too often in practice, a natural side-effect of our modern lives, it seems (Winston & Maimes, 2007).

Immunity

Another side-effect is lowered immunity. Although ashwagandha isn't effective in killing the bacteria or viruses that are the cause of most colds, it does help us to battle against these by supporting immunity. It's probably best used preventatively than during a cold (Winston & Maimes, 2007).

Digestion

Though I haven't used it for this myself the herb is wonderful for malnutrition (Winston & Maimes, 2007). Not a surprise for a herb that builds up energy such as this.

Endocrine

Ashwagandha is mostly used as an adaptogen where it helps to calm the system. However, I have found that for some who are particularly run down even ashwagandha can be too stimulating! For them it's best to start with a long course of nervines and tonics instead (Winston & Maimes, 2007).

My particular favourite use of ashwagandha is its ability to improve the quality of eggs in a woman. To do this you need to consume it for 3 months before trying to get pregnant, as it takes 3 months to take full effect, brilliant for supporting people through IVF.

Safety Considerations

Possible sensitivity to its plant family; solanacea (deadly night-shade family). May not suit people with hyperthyroidism.

—— Zingiber officinale (ginger) ——

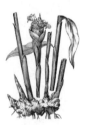

Names: n/a

Element: Fire

Planet: Mars

Magical uses: good health, protection of physical health

Key words: heat, warmth, enliven, energy

Tissue state: depression, constriction and atrophy

Qualities: diffusive, stimulating, warm

Actions: anti inflammatory, carminative, antispasmodic, expectorant, vasodilator, anti cholesterol, circulatory stimulant, antiemetic, diaphoretic

Physical uses: nausea, flatulence, colitis, IBS, diarrhoea, peptic ulcers, loss of appetite, cold and flu, pneumonia, post nasal drip, swollen glands, phlegm on the chest, dry ticklish cough, cold peripheries, hiccup, brain fog, weakness, jet lag, atherosclerosis, period pain, stagnant blood, strength in labour

Emotional uses: adds inner fire and passion to despondent people

Parts used: root

Known constituents: phenolic compounds, gingerols, mucilage, volatile oils

Legend and tradition

Traditionally ginger was preserved by boiling in sugar and turned into crystalised ginger. The syrup that the ginger was soaked in used to be fermented and turned into liquor called "cool drink". Though I'm sure it was anything but cooling. It is said to be native to Asia where it has a long history of medicinal use and didn't make it to Britain until we were able to import it, becoming well known here by the eleventh century (Grieves, 1992).

Medicinal uses

Immunity

The warming effect of ginger is far stronger than cinnamon. It is excellent for bringing on a sweat to cool a fever. But also helps lessen swollen glands, pneumonia and postnasal drip (Grieves, 1992).

Cardiovascular

As a circulatory stimulant the herb helps to clear stagnant blood, bringing blood where it needs to be, usually, towards the peripheries. But for some, ginger can help bring blood flow to the uterus and help with painful and light but clotted periods (Brooke, 1992).

Digestion

Ginger has been highly researched for its usefulness in treating nausea. No matter the cause, ginger seems to help and is perfectly safe during pregnancy. It is helpful where coldness is creating slow motility in the digestion leading to flatulence, IBS and loss of appetite. But, ironically, it can help with inflammatory diseases like colitis! (Brooke, 1992)

Reproduction

The heat of ginger helps to give strength during labour, but I'd also use it to give some fire to someone who is sick (Brooke, 1992).

Safety Considerations

Don't use with kidney disease

See overpage for herbal uses chart » »

HERBAL USES CHART	Heavy period	Light period	Short cycle	Long cycle	Irregular cycle	Period pain	Menstrual migraines	Hormonal spots	Sore breasts	PMS
Alfalfa (pg. 196)		X	X	X	X					
Ashwagandha (pg. 238)	X	X	X	X	X					X
Burdock root (pg. 168)		X	X				X	X	X	
Chamomile (pg. 178)					X		X			X
Cinnamon (pg. 181)		X	X			X	X			
Cleavers (pg. 188)								X	X	
Dandelion leaf (pg. 228)									X	
Dandelion root (pg. 227)	X	X	X	X	X	X		X	X	
Elderberry (pg. 220)										
Elderflower (pg. 222)										X
Elecampane (pg. 193)										X
Ginger (pg. 240)		X	X			X	X			
Hawthorn (pg. 185)	X	X	X	X	X					X
Hyssop (pg. 191)										
Lemonbalm (pg. 198)	X	X	X	X	X	X	X			X
Lime blossom (pg. 231)	X	X	X	X	X	X	X			X
Liquorice (pg. 190)	X	X	X	X	X					X
Marigold (pg. 173)	X	X	X	X	X			X	X	
Marshmallow (pg. 165)						X				
Nettle (pg. 235)	X	X	X	X	X				X	
Oat (pg. 171)	X	X	X	X	X	X	X			X
Orange blossom (pg. 183)	X	X	X	X	X	X	X			X
Passionflower (pg. 206)						X	X			X
Peppermint (pg. 201)	X			X	X					
Raspberry leaf (pg. 218)	X				X					
Rhodiola (pg. 208)	X	X	X	X	X	X	X			X
Rose (pg. 210)		X	X							
Rosemary (pg. 214)		X	X							
Shepherd's purse (pg. 176)	X									
Skullcap (pg. 224)	X	X	X	X	X	X	X			X
Spearmint (pg. 204)	X			X	X					
Thyme (pg. 229)								X		

PMDD	Ovulation pain	Fatigue	Anxiety	Depression	Insomnia	Cold extremities	Hot flushes	Low immunity	Night sweats	Digestive complaints	Cystitis	Infertility	Thrush
		X						X				X	
X		X	X	X	X			X				X	
										X			
X			X	X	X					X			
	X	X		X		X		X		X			
								X			X		
							X		X				
	X			X			X		X	X			
								X			X		
X		X	X	X	X			X					
X		X	X	X	X			X					
	X	X				X							
X		X	X	X	X							X	
		X					X				X		
X	X		X	X	X					X		X	X
X	X		X	X	X		X		X	X		X	
X		X	X	X	X		X	X	X	X		X	
							X		X		X		X
										X	X		X
		X	X	X	X						X	X	
X	X	X	X	X	X		X		X			X	
X	X	X	X	X	X								
X	X		X	X	X							X	
				X			X		X	X			
	X											X	X
X	X	X	X	X	X		X	X	X			X	
X		X	X	X		X		X		X	X	X	
X		X	X	X		X		X		X	X	X	
X	X		X		X							X	
							X		X	X			
							X			X		X	

Conclusion

We are taught through our culture and science that our ovaries are out to get us. I hope that this book has given you all you need to remember the truth: your ovaries *love* you. Your whole body does for that matter. It's here to help you, not punish you.

I've given you the most up-to-date science available when it comes to your hormones, and I hope it has freed you from the dogma of "female-body-as-curse"; as it did for me so many years ago.

Because, when we keep on seeing uniquely female experiences as "all bad" we continue a tradition of self-hatred dating back thousands of years, starting with the idea that women are of the devil, and therefore inferior.

Modern science can help us to understand our bodies for ourselves, rather than dictating a body image based on religious or sexist bias as it has in the past. We aren't completely free of those patriarchal beliefs, as they are so ingrained, but we can use the facts in this book to spread the good word and *embrace our ovaries!*

References

Azziz, R. et.al. (2004) The Prevalence and Features of the Polycistic Ovary Sydrome in an Unselected Population. JCEM. Volume 89, Issue 6, 1 June 2004, Pages 2745–2749.

Bartram, (1995) *Bartram's Encyclopaedia of Herbal Medicine*. Robinson: England.

Brandt, A. (1985) *No Magic Bullet: A Social History of Venereal Disease in the United States Since 1880*. New York: Oxford University Press.

Brooke, E. (1992) *The Woman's Book of Herbs*. The Women's Press limited: London.

Collins, S. et.al. (2013). *Oxford Handbook of Obstetrics and Gynaecology*. 3rd ed. OUP: Oxford.

Crockett, L. (2018). *Healing Our Hormones, Healing Our Lives*. John Hunt Publishing: England.

Culpeper, N. (1979) *Culpeper's Complete Herbal*. Facsimile Edition: England.

Davis, N. (2017) Can an app really provide effective birth control? *The Guardian*. [online] Accessed 12/1/18 from: *https://www.theguardian.com/society/2017/oct/15/can-apps-provide-effective-birth-control-contraception-sexual-freedom.*

Elhag, K., Bahar, A., Mubarak, A. (1988) The effect of a copper intra-uterine contraceptive device on the microbial ecology of the female genital tract. *Journal of Medical Microbiolgy.* Apr;25 (4):245–51. [online] Accessed 5/1/18: https://www.ncbi.nlm.nih. gov/pubmed/3357191.

Endometriosis-uk.org, (2018) *Understanding Endometriosis.* Available from: https://www.endometriosis-uk.org/ understanding-endometriosis [Accessed 5th September 2018].

Ferreira-Poblete, A. (1997) The probability of conception on different days of the cycle with respect to ovulation: An overview. *Advances in Contraception.* 12, (2-3), p.83–95.

Forster, K (2017) Labiaplasty: Vaginal surgery 'world's fastest-growing cosmetic procedure', say plastic surgeons [online] The Independent. Available at: https://www.independent. co.uk/news/health/labiaplasty-vagina-surgery- cosmetic-procedure-plastic-study-international-societ y-aesthetic-plastic-a7837181.html#r3z-addoor [Accessed 27 Nov 2018].

Frizzell, N. (2017) The coil isn't just a great contraceptive, it's a form of resistance for US women. The Guardian, 23 January 2017. [online] accessed 5/1/18: https://www.theguardian.com/ commentisfree/2017/jan/23/contraceptive- american-women-coil-iud-womens-reproductive-rights.

Gov.uk (2015) *Intrauterine contraception: uterine perforation— updated information on risk factors.* [online] Accessed 5/1/18: https://www.gov.uk/drug-safety-update/intrauterine- contraception-uterine-perforation-updated-information-on- risk-factors.

Greenfield, P. (2017) *Half of young people do not use condoms for sex with new partner – poll*. The Guardian. Accessed online: https://www.theguardian.com/society/2017/dec/15/condom-use-survey-sexually-active-young-people-england

Grieves, (1992) The Modern Herbal. 3rd Ed. Tiger Books International: England.

Halbreich, U. et.al. (2003) The prevalence, impairment, impact, and burden of premenstrual dysphoric disorder (PMS/PMDD). *Psychoneroendocrinology*. 28, (3), p.1–23.

Hubacher, D. (2014) Intrauterine devices & infection: Review of the literature. *Indian J Med Res*. 2014 Nov; 140(Suppl 1): S53–S57. [online] Accessed 5/1/18: https://www.ncbi.nlm.nih.gov/pmc/articles/PMC4345753/.

Hughes and Owen (2016) *Weeds in the Heart*. Quintessence Press: England.

Irani, S. (2018) Painful Periods (dysmenorrhea). *Bupa.co.uk*. [online] Accessed 29/1/18: https://www.bupa.co.uk/health-information/womens-health/dysmenorrhoea.

Jonsson. B.1, Landgren, BM., Eneroth, P. (1991) Effects of various IUDs on the composition of cervical mucus. *Contraception*. May;43 (5) :447–58. [online] accessed on 5/1/2018: https://www.ncbi.nlm.nih.gov/pubmed/1914458.

Knight, J. (2016) *The Complete guide to Fertility Awareness*. Routledge: London.

Kumar, P. & Clark, M. (2016) *Kumar and Clark's Clinical Medicine*. 9th Ed. Elsevier: England.

Manisoff, M. (1973) Family planning training for social service: a teaching guide in family planning.

Marsh, K. Et.al. (2010) Effect of a low glycemic index compared with a conventional healthy diet on polycystic ovary syndrome. *The American Journal of Clinical Nutrition*, vol.92:1 p. 83-92, 1 July 2010 [available online] https://doi.org/10.3945/ajcn.2010.29261.

McCulloch, F. (2018) The Pregnenolone Steal: A Closer Look at this Popular Concept. drfionand.com. [online] https://drfion-and.com/2018/03/22/pregnenolone-steal-closer-look-popular-concept/ Accessed 21st December 2018.

Meuleman C, Vandenabeele B, Fieuws S, Spiessens C, Timmerman D, D'Hooghe T. (2009) High prevalence of endometriosis in infertile women with normal ovulation and normospermic partners. *Fertility Sterility* 2009;92(1):68–74.

Murphy, M. (2018) Natural Cycles contraceptive app reported after influx of unwanted pregnancies. The Telegraph. [online] Access 8/3/18 from: https://www.telegraph.co.uk/technology/2018/01/16/natural-cycles-contraceptive-app-reported-influx-unwanted-pregnancies/.

Natural Cycles (2017) How it Works. [online] Accessed 14/1/18 from: https://www.naturalcycles.com/en/contraception/howitworks.

NHS, (2017) Natural Family Planning. NHS [online]. Accessed 15/1/18: https://www.nhs.uk/conditions/contraception/natural-family-planning/?

NIAIAD (2001) The National Institute of Allergy and Infectious Diseases. HIV/AIDS Statistics. Accessed online: http://www.niaid.nih.gov/factsheets/aidsstat.htm

Parewijck, W., Claeys, G., Thiery, M. van Kets, H. (1988) Candidiasis in women fitted with an intrauterine contraceptive device. *British Journal of Obstetrics and Gynaecology*. Apr; 95(4):408–10. [online] Accessed 5/1/18: https://www.ncbi.nlm.nih.gov/pubmed/3382616.

Parry, V. (2005). *Calendar girls*. [online] The Guardian. Available at: https://www.theguardian.com/society/2005/aug/25/health.lifeandhealth [Accessed 27 Nov. 2018].

PFAF.org, (2017) *Inula Helenium*. [available online] http://pfaf.org/user/Plant.aspx?LatinName=Inula+helenium. Accessed 4/5/18.

Radiology Society of North America (2012) Migration of Intrauterine Devices: Radiologic Findings and Implications for Patient Care. RSNA. March-April; 32(2). [online] Accessed 5/1/18 http://pubs.rsna.org/doi/full/10.1148/rg.322115068.

Rogers PA, D'Hooghe TM, Fazleabas A, et al. (2009) Priorities for endometriosis research: recommendations from an international consensus workshop. *Reprodictive Science* 2009;16(4):335–46.

Scott, E (2016) 44% of women can't correctly identify the vagina. [online] The Metro. Available at: https://metro.co.uk/2016/09/02/44-of-women-cant-correctly-identify-the-vagina-6105922/ [Accessed 27 Nov 2018].

Scherwitzly, E. et.al. (2016) Fertility awareness-based mobile application for contraception. *The European Journal of Contraception and Reproductive Health Care*. 21, (3), p.234–241.

Sarner, M (2017) *What comes in 66 sizes and vegan latex? The new generation of condoms*. The Guardian. Availabe from: https://

www.theguardian.com / society / 2017 / oct / 23 / what-comes-66-size-vegan-latex-new-generation-of-condoms [Accessed 24 Oct 2018].

Systeme, P. (1775) Physique et moral de le femme. Paris: Vincent. p.207 Laws, S., Hey, V. & Eagan, A. (1985) *Seeing Red: The politics of premenstrual tension*. Hutchinson and Co. (Publishing) Ltd: Australia.

Taiwo, A., Leite, F., Lucena, G., Barros, M., Silveira, D., Silva, M. and Ferreira, V. (2012) Anxiolytic and antidepressant-like effects of *Melissa officinalis* (lemon balm) extract in rats: Influence of administration and gender. *Indian Journal of Pharmacology*. Mar–Apr; 44(2): 189–192. [Online] Available from: https: / /www.ncbi.nlm.nih.gov / pmc / articles / PMC3326910 / [Accessed: 3rd October 2017].

Trickey, R. (2003) *Women, Hormones, and the Menstrual Cycle*. Allen & Unwin: Australia.

University of California (2015) *The History of the Condom*. Accessed online: http: / /www.soc.ucsb.edu / sexinfo / article / history-condom.

Wilkinson, Tholandi, Ramjez, Rutherford (2002). Nonoxynol-9 spermicide for prevention of vaginally acquired HIV and other sexually transmitted infections: systematic review and meta-analysis of randomised controlled trials including more than 5000 women. The Lancet: *Infectious Diseases*. [Accessed online] Available from: http: / /www.doi.org / 10.1016 / S1473-3099(02)00396-1.

Winston, D., 2007. *Adaptogens*. Inner Traditions / Bear & Co.

Wood, M. (2008) *The Earthwise Herbal: A complete guide to old world medicinal plants.* North Atlantic Books: USA.

Wyss, R. & Bourrit, B. (1986) GYNAKOLOGISCHE RUNDS-CHAU. Nov; 26 Supp 1:18-24. [accessed online] https://www.popline.org/node/350907.

Zhang, J., Feldman, P., Chi, I., Gaston Farr, M. (1992) Risk factors for copper T IUD expulsion: An epidemiologic analysis. *Contraception.* 46(5): 427–433 [online]. Accessed 5/1/18: http://www.sciencedirect.com/science/article/pii/001078249290146K.

Ziegenfuss, T. et.al. (2006) Effects of a Water-Soluble Cinnamon Extract on Body Composition and Features of the Metabolic Syndrome in Pre-Diabetic Men and Women.
Journal of the International Society of Sports Nutrition. 2006, vol.3:45. [available online] https://doi.org/10.1186/1550-2783-3-2-45.